Praise for *The Secret Female Hormone*

"I have long recommended testosterone to those women who require it. Dr. Maupin's updated and thorough approach to this little-known female hormone is simply excellent."

—**Christiane Northrup, MD, OB/GYN,** and *New York Times* best-selling author of *Women's Bodies, Women's Wisdom* and *The Wisdom of Menopause*

"*The Secret Female Hormone* unveils the missing link for many women over 40 who are suffering from symptoms such as low libido, fatigue, insomnia, loss of muscle mass, and an increase in belly fat—despite the perfect diet and exercise regime. Every woman should read this book!"

—**Dr. Natasha Turner,** naturopathic doctor and author of *The Hormone Diet, The Supercharged Hormone Diet,* and *The Carb Sensitivity Plan*

"*The Secret Female Hormone* is a must read for women today! Dr. Maupin and Mr. Newcomb have brought to light the importance of testosterone for many women struggling with low libido. Hormones should always be evaluated in unity, and testosterone is almost always overlooked. The authors tell the truth about how hormone imbalances truly affect women—not only their energy, their vitality, and their libido but also their family relationships and self-esteem. This book will be a resource for women for years to come!"

—**Marcelle Pick, MSN, OB/GYN NP,** owner of Women to Women and author of *Is It Me or My Hormones?* and *The Core Balance Diet*

THE SECRET FEMALE HORMONE

Hay House Titles of Related Interest

THE
SECRET FEMALE
HORMONE

HOW **TESTOSTERONE REPLACEMENT**
CAN CHANGE YOUR LIFE

KATHY C. MAUPIN MD
WITH BRETT NEWCOMB

HAY HOUSE

Carlsbad, California • New York City • London • Sydney
Johannesburg • Vancouver • Hong Kong • New Delhi

First published and distributed in the United Kingdom by:
Hay House UK Ltd, Astley House, 33 Notting Hill Gate, London W11 3JQ
Tel: +44 (0)20 3675 2450; Fax: +44 (0)20 3675 2451
www.hayhouse.co.uk

Published and distributed in the United States of America by:
Hay House Inc., PO Box 5100, Carlsbad, CA 92018-5100
Tel: (1) 760 431 7695 or (800) 654 5126
Fax: (1) 760 431 6948 or (800) 650 5115
www.hayhouse.com

Published and distributed in Australia by:
Hay House Australia Ltd, 18/36 Ralph St, Alexandria NSW 2015
Tel: (61) 2 9669 4299; Fax: (61) 2 9669 4144
www.hayhouse.com.au

Published and distributed in the Republic of South Africa by:
Hay House SA (Pty) Ltd, PO Box 990, Witkoppen 2068
Tel/Fax: (27) 11 467 8904
www.hayhouse.co.za

Published and distributed in India by:
Hay House Publishers India, Muskaan Complex, Plot No.3, B-2,
Vasant Kunj, New Delhi 110 070
Tel: (91) 11 4176 1620; Fax: (91) 11 4176 1630
www.hayhouse.co.in

Distributed in Canada by:
Raincoast Books, 2440 Viking Way, Richmond, B.C. V6V 1N2
Tel: (1) 604 448 7100; Fax: (1) 604 270 7161; www.raincoast.com

Indexer: Jay Kreider • *Cover design:* Patricia Martin-Owen • *Interior design:* Nick C. Welch • *Image on page 238:* Romondo Davis • *All other images:* Eric W. Wilson

A catalogue record for this book is available from the British Library.

ISBN: 978-1-78180-178-9

Printed and bound in Great Britain by TJ International Ltd, Padstow, Cornwall.

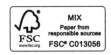

MIX
Paper from
responsible sources
FSC
www.fsc.org   FSC® C013056

The greatest joy of my medical life was delivering miracles to my sisters, my patients, as I shared the moment of childbirth with them . . . until 11 years ago. That is when my calling was redirected, and I discovered a new miracle to share with my sisters. In a mysterious revelation, I uncovered Woman's fountain of youth. I was personally reborn when I replaced a hormone we once had that has been lost in time. Like an archaeologist digging through research and subterfuge, I have unearthed the one hormone that can revive our struggling bodies after age 40. This book is a map for my beloved sisters who have given their lives to their families and to time—so now they can get their lives back!

CONTENTS

PREFACE

The Secret Hormone That Saved My Life

Women love sharing a secret recipe, a stain removal treatment, and other tricks of the female trade. The secret *I* love to share—my "secret ingredient"—is testosterone. This single hormone is the father and mother of all hormones involved in health, reproduction, sexuality, mood, immunity, lean body mass, bone thickness, and mental clarity. Testosterone is important not only for maintaining general health in women but for treating a wide variety of ailments that most doctors ascribe to simple aging. In fact, these symptoms are *not* the result of simple aging; they are a singular condition that testosterone can in fact reverse completely, helping women recapture the youthfulness and vibrancy of their early 30s.

Currently, testosterone is considered a "male hormone," which means that traditional hormone replacement for women does not include it. And while it is true that men must have much higher levels of testosterone in their blood than women do in order to be healthy, many people are surprised to learn that testosterone is just as essential to women's well-being as it is to men's.

Unfortunately, testosterone's value to women is something of a secret because mainstream medicine has not approved its use for women. The reasons for this have less to do with health care than with gender politics. Historically, the U.S. medical profession and the FDA, both of which are generally run by men, have refused to approve for use by women many drugs that have testosterone in them while approving them for treatment of male sexual problems.

Yet I'm here to tell you that testosterone can change your life; it changed mine.

My trip through hormonal hell began when I was in my early 40s. Long before menopause, I began a free fall into a state of debilitation. I was busy taking care of a husband, a daughter, and a medical practice, and I was involved in many charities, organizations, and political groups. With so much to do, I hardly had time to notice the differences in my mind, body, and soul. I suffered overwhelming fatigue, insomnia, and mood changes. I gained weight, lost interest in sex, and experienced severe PMS (premenstrual syndrome) and migraines, and my personality became flat. Along the way, I lost sight of my own well-being. I did what many do under such stress: I limited my activities to home and office and cut everything else out of my life.

Before these symptoms began to affect me, I was considered the go-to hormone expert in St. Louis. Some even referred to me as the "hormone queen"! I was already a fan of bio-identical hormones, which are natural because they are made from plants and identical to human hormones, so I treated myself with pure progesterone. Voilà! For a brief time I was back to my normal self!

Unfortunately, though, it didn't last; I found myself severely limited again. I tried everything I knew, including replacing bio-identical sublingual tablets, vaginal suppositories, and patches and creams with estradiol and progesterone. Nothing worked. I was completely exhausted, unable to sleep, and waking up in the middle of the night with racing thoughts. I gained 20 pounds and was continually depressed. I was too tired to work out, which I had routinely done since college, too swollen to put on my wedding ring, and couldn't sleep at all. The insomnia was the worst of it because it led to fatigue, crankiness, a craving for carbs, and other unhealthy habits. After I completely lost my sex drive, I viewed myself in an asexual way . . . a very subtle change that only my husband noticed. I looked and felt old.

Progesterone obviously was not the answer—something else was missing. I tried conventional hormone treatment and every bio-identical hormone replacement available, yet nothing in my hormone queen's little black bag could help me! It's hard to believe now, but at just 43 years old, I *hoped* I could still be productive. Desperate for help, I sought evaluation by several internists. They all said I was healthy, just "getting old" or "being lazy." Some even suggested I was crazy and referred me to psychiatrists, all of whom deemed me sane. Most of these physicians talked to me in the exact same way, as if this were all in my head.

Unwilling to accept the doctors' diagnoses—or lack of one—I researched the problem as best I could for myself. I began to suspect that it was not a group of unrelated symptoms secondary to aging but some sort of "condition" or "syndrome" related to hormone deprivation. Unfortunately I found very few articles in the OB/GYN literature to help me. I then went back to basic medicine and reviewed the physiology of hormonal balance, but because I did not look for articles specifically about testosterone and did not look in medical literature outside of the specialties of obstetrics and gynecology, I continued to flounder.

I ultimately concluded that conventional medicine had failed to comprehensively tackle this issue that is so crucial to a majority of women. I also knew I was not alone; I had tried many replacements with conventional and bio-identical hormones of the transdermal, sublingual, and cream types with other patients, who, like me, felt only slightly better in the end.

Throughout my research, I continued to feel progressively worse in every area. Like many people, I also had other issues: in my case, progressively worsening endometriosis that was going to require a hysterectomy and removal of my ovaries. And, as many other female doctors do, I waited until the pain was so bad that I could not walk. I eventually was forced to face the devastating possibility that I would have to reduce my commitments or perhaps resign my practice altogether. I finally underwent the surgery, hoping that all my symptoms were the result of chronic pain.

My hysterectomy was not a normal surgery. I was given nine liters of fluid to resuscitate me afterward, which caused me to go into cardiac failure. I was entering ARDS, a severe lung malfunction, and was on a respirator when I woke up long before anticipated. I could tell I was in the ICU because I recognized it; I had done my residency at the same hospital more than 20 years earlier. I was alone, with hands and feet restrained so I could not move. The tube in my throat made me feel like I was choking, and I could not reach the call button to summon a nurse, so I kicked my legs until the cardiac monitor went off and two nurses came in.

I struggled to communicate, but it was as if I wasn't even there. The nurses didn't acknowledge me, never looked me in the eye, instead they talked quietly to each other.

That was when I hit bottom: the worst hour of my life. I prayed to die because I did not want to live as a cardiac cripple.

Then, suddenly, the most amazing thing happened. The stress of struggling to breathe won out, and I had a near-death experience in the ICU. The serenity and peace I found in the place where I awakened was so wonderful that I wanted to stay there. But I was sent back because, I was told, there was "special work" for me to do.

A dear friend miraculously appeared at my bedside. He unstrapped my hands, removed the tube from my throat, and gave me a pen to write with, which allowed me to communicate and describe what I needed. At that moment everything reversed, and I was home in two days, alive and well.

After months of intense recovery, battling the same problems I described earlier, I was still searching for answers when Gina, a nurse I had known forever, recommended I set up a meeting with her brother, Dr. Gino Tutera. Gino had been replacing hormones with bio-identical subdermal testosterone pellets for more than 20 years, achieving remarkable results. When he treated me, the results were nothing short of miraculous.

Gino taught me about the importance of testosterone in women's lives. A hormone that we aren't even aware of could cure all the things that ailed me? It seemed too good to be true. But it wasn't! Implanting natural bio-identical estradiol and testosterone pellets and using Armour Thyroid (natural pig thyroid) brought me back to health and youth! I slept straight through the night the first time I took the pellets, and then every other symptom disappeared! Almost magically, I was my old energetic, healthy, sexual self again.

I have now used bio-identical testosterone pellets for 11 years. I have been free of migraines, and I sleep like a baby. I am down to my predisaster weight, and I feel great! All the symptoms that had been haunting me—weight gain, loss of libido, fatigue, and an inability to think quickly—have been resolved. I have my life back because of BioBalance pellets. Since my own treatment began, I've been trained in administering these same replacement pellets, and I am passionate about spreading the word.

My excitement about replacing lost testosterone with bio-identical forms has grown each day since I started replacement therapy myself and began treating women over 40 with testosterone. The results have been phenomenal: literally no other treatment in medicine has a 95 percent success rate in resolving a condition and all its symptoms. It is remarkable to me that I can sustain this rate of success in my practice, but it has been proven again and again when my patients return glowing with health, self-esteem, and beauty.

I can now look back with gratitude upon my health crisis, even though it was an extremely difficult time for me, emotionally and physically. The experience opened the door for thousands of women to receive effective treatment with bio-identical testosterone.

I now know that my "special work"—my ultimate calling—is to help treat and cure the pain and distress of all who suffer from testosterone deficiency and deserve this quality-of-life-saving treatment. I'm here to help women become whole again and reclaim their lives. I've written this book for all women, and for *you*.

Kathy C. Maupin, MD

INTRODUCTION

Have you ever wondered why we get old? There are many theories out there. Generally they blame the environment or toxins but do not explain what triggers the process of aging. The answer is hidden deep in the medical literature of the specialty called endocrinology, and it comes down to one hormone—testosterone. In women, testosterone is produced by the ovaries, and production begins to decrease at around the age of 40; this is the first trigger for aging. Then other hormones follow suit, reducing their production in response to the drop in testosterone, and so we slide almost unconsciously into premature old age.

In this book, we will explain the whys and hows of this process, but more important, the *cure* for testosterone deficiency and the symptoms of aging. We will also pay close attention to the reasons for the U.S. medical community's stance on testosterone replacement: Why does it fully embrace this treatment for men but not women? Why hasn't your doctor considered this replacement in response to your complaints? There is a reason the American, British, and Canadian medical establishments have buried testosterone replacement for women, and you will learn why you are only now hearing of this "secret treatment."

KNOWLEDGE IS POWER

When you talk to a medical professional about hormone replacement choices, the more you know, the better. Almost all women know to ask about the benefits and risks of a treatment a doctor proposes for them, but most don't know enough to ask about the benefits and risks of *not* taking a treatment like testosterone! This book offers both the pros and cons of doing so and discusses why the risks associated with refusing treatment for hormone deprivation are significant and, for most people, far outweigh the risks of accepting it. Remember, a choice not to do something is still a choice! It, too, has consequences. Know what they are.

KATHY MAUPIN, MD: WHO I AM—MY TRAINING AND BACKGROUND

As a board-certified obstetrician and gynecologist, I have practiced OB/GYN medicine for more than 25 years and delivered thousands of babies. I am currently an antiaging physician, dedicated to treating women with the secret hormone, testosterone, something we all need after the age of 40, in the safest and most natural way possible.

For many years I had been listening to my patients' complaints about exhaustion, lack of libido, belly fat, migraines, and other symptoms as they approached or experienced menopause. All too often I heard the simple, plaintive cry, "Doctor, what is wrong with me?"

It is not a casual question. It is a question almost always uttered in desperation. Until a few years ago, I did not know the answer and I had to tell my patients so.

This book is for all the women who have experienced the drastic and debilitating effects of hormonal imbalance as they approach midlife, even before menopause, and have not received help through conventional medicine.

I was one of those women. I know the desperation that sets in after many frustrating visits to doctors who do not understand the problem or the solution. So I can tell you firsthand that life does not have to end after 40! I want to share the secret of testosterone with you so you can live the next half of your life with energy, health, and joy.

I know that finding the right treatment is difficult for women who are not trained as doctors, and I understand the dilemma of experiencing symptoms that no one believes or will help try to solve. It is a blessing that I was a physician when I experienced the symptoms of testosterone deprivation; I had the training to find an answer on my own. Now I can pass along what I learned and help *all women* look for and request the right treatment to make them whole again. I very much want to reach women who are suffering from hormone loss, in the hope of helping them regain their health through a novel, safe, and effective hormone replacement regimen.

I can't tell you how fulfilling my medical practice is now! I am able to sustain more than a 95 percent success rate for my patients with hormone replacement using the safest type (bio-identical pellets) while including the critical and often forgotten female hormone testosterone. This has led me to dedicate *all* of my efforts to my BioBalance hormone replacement practice, and I no longer practice the traditional medical specialties of obstetrics or gynecology.

The satisfaction I derive from helping women recover their lives, and from intervening in ways that restore them to vigor and health, is inexpressible, but it inspired me to write this book about my journey of knowledge and the changes in my own life. I hope that my experience will help others discover what I now know, not only from personal experience but from helping literally thousands of women journey back to health.

This book is the fulfillment of that hope.

Before I began this project, I knew I needed someone with different skills to help me. Good health care involves not only the physical but the psychological as well, so I enlisted the help of my good friend and professional colleague Brett Newcomb.

BRETT NEWCOMB, MA, LPC: WHO I AM—MY TRAINING AND BACKGROUND

I have spent 30 years working as a family therapist. During that time, I have met with many people struggling with what I thought were psychologically caused and stress-induced issues. Over the years, I have learned that many psychological or emotional difficulties are also physical ones. Through the opportunity to work with good physicians such as Dr. Maupin, I have learned much about the overlapping and interweaving of the physical and the psychological.

I have collaborated with Kathy for years, consulting with clients of mine who are also her patients. Together we have worked to find the optimal interface of behavioral and physiological treatments to help our patients have the best quality of life possible as they age.

We first began working together because we had a mutual patient. Sandra was having marital problems and thought she might have depression. I always ask clients who are suffering from depression to have a medical exam to rule out any physical causes. After Sandra saw Kathy, she gave us both permission to communicate about her case. As our work progressed, we determined that Sandra was not suffering from depression after all, but that her issues were related to a lack of libido resulting from a low testosterone level, and this affected her marriage. Her husband, Bill, was 53 and still wanted sex several times a week. Sandra felt like her sex drive was depleted. She still loved Bill, but she just had no sexual desire. I worked with Bill and Sandra on their ability to communicate, and Dr. Maupin worked on testosterone replacement for Sandra. Bill and Sandra experienced a revival of their sex lives and a strengthening of their marriage, and Dr. Maupin and I were off and running to collaborate with other patients whenever appropriate!

We have written this book together in much the same way we collaborate in our work with clients. Kathy focuses on her experience and the medical science she knows and uses to help patients. I add insights and recommendations from my own clinical perspective, concentrating on the communication skills that help people reality test what is going on in their lives and decide on a course of action to make their relationships better. These skills are to a large extent volitional. Once you learn them, you must decide to actually use them. I will provide both the tools and encouragement you need to utilize the information that both of us offer in this book.

How This Book Is Organized

It is important that you understand how this book is set up so you can get the most out of it. We've written it to explain why the medical profession should acknowledge the existence of a newly discovered syndrome in women: TDS, or testosterone deficiency syndrome. We hope this will lead to better treatment and healing for women whose complaints have long been ignored by mainstream medicine. Ultimately, we describe the treatment we believe works best for the greatest number of women. As an individual, you will need to assess what we have provided in terms of your own unique situation.

Our primary focus in this book is testosterone because it is the *central hormone* in the aging process, and understanding what reduced production of it brings about is important for *all* women. Our other hormones, progesterone and estrogen—specifically the estrogen called estradiol—are also important, but these are already well known to women and you can find many books and resources that deal with their role in aging. But until very recently, testosterone has not been thought of as a woman's hormone, even though it's an essential part of our makeup. If you're like many women and you suffer from TDS, you *need* testosterone. You may or may not need progesterone and/or estrogen, but you do need testosterone.

In Part I of the book, we identify and explain what TDS is. We underscore the importance of testosterone in the lives of women, discuss the history of TDS, explain why TDS isn't acknowledged as a woman's problem, and most important, offer an easy and informative questionnaire to help you determine whether you have or might develop TDS. We also introduce you to the "aging cascade" as a whole, and each stage of women's aging: testosterone loss, progesterone loss, and estradiol loss (also known as menopause).

Part II breaks down the three female hormones involved in the aging cascade that is triggered by the loss of testosterone. As a result of these changes, our hormone-dependent systems begin to deteriorate and age us. We pay special attention to sex and libido as they relate to your hormones—namely testosterone. In order to understand sexual dysfunction, you need to understand healthy sexual function. The presence or absence of testosterone is the origin of libido and the sex drive.

We will take an in-depth look at the symptoms that indicate testosterone deficiency so you can more thoroughly understand this condition. We'll also examine the long-term illnesses that are caused by the loss of testosterone. Throughout, you will find questionnaires to help you determine if you are suffering from the loss of these hormones, along with advice for what to do if you are.

Toward the end of Part II, we'll examine the second and third ovarian hormones—progesterone and estrogen. Two hormones, testosterone and estrogen, are whole-body hormones important throughout our lives, required for balancing the hormonal system. During childbearing years, there is a third full-body hormone present: progesterone. This is necessary to balance the extreme fluctuations in estrogen that are possible. After menopause, if we do not have a uterus, or if we are using a Mirena IUD, we do not need progesterone. When we are given estrogen replacement, progesterone is necessary only to regulate bleeding in the uterus. It is no longer a whole-body regulating hormone.

Because of testosterone's importance as a female hormone, it is central to this book. Information about estrogen and progesterone, while important, is already widely available; we will address these two hormones in a single chapter. Yet you will find helpful questionnaires concerning all three of these hormones, including symptoms of deficiency and risks and benefits of replacement.

In Part III, we discuss the risks and benefits of choosing to either replace your hormones or do nothing at all. You will find an overview of the physical, financial, and emotional risks and benefits for each decision you must make. All of this leads to the final chapter, which will help you decide which hormones to replace and which type of replacement will work best for you.

This book presents you with a road map to determine which of these hormone losses you may suffer from, and to decide on a course of action if you do. It offers a complete description of the costs, benefits, and protocols involved in getting back on your feet. We want you to regain the vim, vigor, and vitality of your youth and live the remainder of your life as a healthy, capable, vibrant woman.

PART I

TESTOSTERONE AND AGING

CHAPTER 1

Do You Have Testosterone Deficiency Syndrome?

Testosterone is a hormone that affects every system of the body. As a result, a lack of it causes global symptoms that are hard to diagnose, including fatigue and depression. There are so many causes for these problems that doctors have trouble knowing where to begin investigating.

Because testosterone loss is a slow process, it often sneaks up on women. They may assume that they changed something in their life or altered their diet or are under undue stress instead of suffering from a medical problem. Most of our patients cannot even pinpoint the *year* their symptoms started unless they had an abrupt loss of their ovaries. To make diagnosis even more difficult, the symptoms of testosterone loss can act like chameleons, seeming like many other medical, emotional, or psychiatric illnesses instead of the deficiency of a single hormone.

Also, to be able to diagnose an illness, a doctor must be taught its symptoms so he or she can consider whether the symptoms fit that pattern. In the case of testosterone deficiency, most doctors do not even know it is a women's illness, which makes it impossible to diagnose (see Chapter 2 for more information on this).

Because we have taken care of thousands of women with this syndrome and have witnessed both the symptoms and the timing of their onset, we have the advantage of experience. We have investigated each symptom and found the research that ties testosterone deficiency with each one. We have found a relationship between the age at which symptoms commonly appear and the situations that trigger diminished testosterone production. Information such as this serves as the basis for the questionnaires we developed to help you determine whether you have TDS.

SELF-ASSESSMENT TOOLS FOR DIAGNOSING TESTOSTERONE DEFICIENCY SYNDROME

Diagnosing a disease of any kind is a complicated process that includes interviewing, physically examining, and testing a patient. The first step is to look at the patient and note her age, weight, and height and whether she looks older or younger than her age, as well as many other tasks that doctors learn to accomplish in the first minute or two of an office visit. The second step involves inquiring about symptoms and their timing and severity. Following that, the doctor performs medical testing (such as blood tests, X-rays, or noting weight changes) to affirm that the diagnosis is correct.

We have adapted this diagnostic process for this book, substituting questionnaires for physician interviews. These questionnaires will tell you whether you are a candidate for laboratory testing and treatment by a physician.

The first questionnaire investigates whether you fit into the age and risk group that can possibly have TDS. Place a check mark next to any statements that apply to you.

- ❏ I am over 38 years old.
- ❏ I have had my ovaries removed.
- ❏ I went through premature menopause before the age of 38.

❏   My ovaries were exposed to radiation while
     undergoing cancer treatment.

*If you checked any of the previous statements, you fit the age and
ovarian status for testosterone deficiency and may have TDS. Now go
on to the next questionnaire.*

The second questionnaire lists the *most common symptoms of
TDS.* Not everyone with TDS has all of these symptoms, but most
women who have testosterone deficiency have at least a few of
them. Place a check mark next to any statements that apply to you.

❏   I have lost my sex drive.
❏   I have had orgasms in the past but can no longer
     have an orgasm, or it is more difficult.
❏   I have more fatigue than before I was 38.
❏   My motivation is gone. I don't feel like doing
     anything!
❏   I have insomnia.
❏   I wake up in the middle of the night and can't go
     back to sleep.
❏   I do not feel rested when I wake up in the morning.
❏   I have a new diagnosis of anxiety and/or depression
     that I did not have before age 38.
❏   I have developed migraine headaches since age 38.
❏   I have gained weight, especially in my belly.
❏   I have decreased exercise stamina.
❏   My muscles are getting smaller, and I am not as
     strong.
❏   My height has decreased.
❏   I have osteopenia or osteoporosis.
❏   I can't remember the names of things, people, or
     places anymore.

- ❏ I have difficulty solving problems and getting organized.
- ❏ I have developed dry eyes that cause me to use medicine or see an eye doctor.
- ❏ I have multiple joint aches, such as arthritis.
- ❏ My knees and hips hurt when I exercise or put any weight on them.
- ❏ I have been diagnosed with an autoimmune disease (MS, rheumatoid arthritis, lupus, scleroderma) after the age of 38.
- ❏ I have lost my balance.
- ❏ My skin is thin and saggy.
- ❏ I look old.
- ❏ I have lost my joy for living. I no longer have a sense of well-being.

Total number of check marks on Symptom Questionnaire = _____

If you answered yes to four or more of the symptoms of TDS, or yes to loss of sex drive and two other symptoms, you probably have TDS.

The third step of diagnosis is medical testing. You may have had blood tests to check your levels of testosterone and other hormones, as well as lab tests to evaluate your general health, and the last questionnaire of this section involves the results of those blood tests that indicate TDS. Most women have abnormal testosterone levels if they have TDS, so the first two blood tests are the most important. However, there are other physiological changes that occur in response to TDS. If you are menstruating, be sure to have your blood drawn in the morning during the first seven days after your period begins to obtain reliable results.

Testosterone Blood Levels for Young, Healthy Women (day 1–7 of cycle)
Total testosterone = 30 ng/dl–60 ng/dl
Free testosterone > 10 pg/ml
Testosterone peaks in the blood day 13–14 of the menstrual cycle

Total testosterone is measured in ng/dl (nanograms per deciliter). Free testosterone is measured in pg/ml (picograms per milliliter). Please ask your doctor for these blood test results. If you have not had these tests yet, please leave this questionnaire until after you have had your blood tests and received the results.

❏ Total testosterone below 30 ng/dl
❏ Free (active) testosterone below 7–10 pg/ml, depending on the lab

At least one of these low testosterone levels is required for you to be diagnosed as having TDS. The most important is the free testosterone because it is the form of the hormone that is active and relates most closely to the symptoms you are experiencing.

Other Blood Tests That Relate to Low Testosterone

❏ Elevated total cholesterol
❏ Elevated LDL cholesterol
❏ Elevated triglycerides
❏ Decreased IGF-1 (growth hormone), less than 150 ng/ml
❏ Elevated luteinizing hormone (LH) greater than 10–16 u/l (units per liter), depending on the lab

If your blood tests display any of these results, you may be able to normalize any of them by replacing testosterone with *a nonoral form of testosterone.*

OTHER CAUSES OF LOW TESTOSTERONE

It is important to note that even if you have had positive results on the preceding questionnaires, the cause of your TDS may not be age related or secondary to failure of your ovaries. This is an important issue your doctor should think about before giving you a solid diagnosis: what else could it be?

Aging is the most common cause of testosterone deficiency, but low testosterone can also be caused by external sources, long before age-related deterioration, or at any time after 40.

Innocently prescribed medications are a major cause of loss of testosterone. These medications are often necessary to treat an appropriate diagnosis but have the side effect of decreasing free testosterone and increasing all of the symptoms of TDS. They include:

- Antidepressants that increase serotonin and decrease sex drive
- Antihypertensives (blood pressure medication) that decrease sexual response and free testosterone
- Birth control pills
- Cholesterol-lowering medication (the statins)
- Evista
- Lupron therapy for endometriosis
- Oral estrogens
- Oral or intramuscular steroids (e.g., Medrol dose pack, prednisone, and hydrocortisone)
- Provera Oral (a synthetic progestin)
- Tamoxifen, which binds testosterone

Anticholesterol Drugs and Testosterone

Since heart disease causes the most deaths in both men and women in the United States, cholesterol-lowering medicine is, by volume, one of the most frequently prescribed medicines in the country. This applies to both men and women. Drugs for high cholesterol can decrease the level of free testosterone in your body, because testosterone is actually made from cholesterol.

Taking cholesterol-lowering medication immediately decreases the production of testosterone and many other hormones.

The medical community is continually reassessing and readjusting its opinion of how much cholesterol in the bloodstream is acceptable. For years the standard of total cholesterol was thought to be less than 220; now the number has dropped to less than 200. For LDL (the "bad cholesterol") the number was recommended to be less than 150 and is now below 130. These numbers are measurements of the dangerous cholesterols that contribute to heart disease.

One form of cholesterol is protective against heart disease, and that number should be greater than 45. A physician has to determine risk/benefit ratio because cholesterol-lowering drugs lower both good and bad forms of cholesterol. Because medicine operates on a triage principle, many doctors focus on the life-threatening issue of heart disease and do not get to the overall quality-of-life issues of libido and sexual happiness. As a doctor, I must ask the question "Why is the impact of cholesterol medicine on testosterone rarely discussed?" If doctors informed patients that decreasing their risk for heart disease would mean not having sex, most of my patients would choose not to take cholesterol medication!

Many doctors advocate for patient participation in medical decision making, yet they tend as a group not to ask their patients about this issue—because they think patients will make the wrong choice! Kathy tries to walk the fine line of helping her patients be good medical consumers, educating them regarding lifestyle choices, and informing them of medicines and their results. This is a time-consuming practice, and not every medical professional has the luxury of sufficient time.

Medications aren't the only factors that contribute to a decrease in testosterone levels in women. Medical conditions such as diabetes and Addison's disease (adrenal failure) can cause low testosterone levels at any age. Even oral estrogens given to treat menopause can bind up testosterone very effectively, making it inactive. (Remember, free testosterone improves libido and makes restoring your sex drive possible.)

If you have one of these conditions and take a medication that lowers your testosterone, it would be reasonable to ask your doctor to change medications or hold the medication (some cannot be held, so don't stop them against your doctor's instructions) and repeat the testosterone blood test. If it normalizes, you have a choice: you can (a) change or adjust your medication dosage or (b) replace testosterone in the safest way to supplement the level in your blood and leave your medications as they are.

Remember: the most common causes of TDS are aging, menopause, and removal of the ovaries, which of course cannot be reversed. The removal of the adrenal glands or part of the pituitary gland can also cause an acute decrease in testosterone production, leading to a full spectrum of symptoms arising from TDS. These are nonreversible but can be treated with testosterone replacement.

So, do you think you might have testosterone deficiency syndrome? If so, read on to find out why this reason for your symptoms has been so hard to find and how to treat your symptoms in a way that is ideal for you.

CHAPTER 2

WHY TESTOSTERONE DEFICIENCY IS NOT ACKNOWLEDGED AS A WOMAN'S DISEASE

Cheryl sat down in Kathy's office, sighed loudly, and said, "Before we start, I have to tell you that I read your story. You had all the symptoms I was experiencing! I was so relieved that I put my head on my kitchen table and cried! All I could think was, *I'm not crazy after all!*"

Like so many other patients, Cheryl had come to feel like she had been invaded, body and soul, by a whole raft of symptoms, including loss of libido, weight gain, insomnia, fatigue, depression, loss of muscle, dry eyes, and migraine headaches. The symptoms kept piling up at an accelerating rate, and despite all the doctors she consulted, she felt ill and looked older than her 45 years.

Unfortunately, despite the fact that she believed that something was wrong—her intuition told her as much—her gynecologist kept telling her that she was simply "getting older" and that there was nothing for her to do but accept it. This false interpretation led her to think she was losing her mind.

Cheryl was a baby boomer. Like most of us of that generation, she believed she could live forever. She couldn't imagine that her healthy, productive life would be over at 45, particularly when her delayed adolescence hadn't ended until her mid-20s. It had never occurred to Cheryl that her quality of life would disappear so soon, especially since she had been very careful to exercise, eat right, and take vitamins and supplements. Just a few years past childbearing age, she felt her life was in many ways over and that her marriage, her family, her job, and her future were all in jeopardy.

Sound familiar?

Why Is the Secret Female Hormone Still a Secret?

There are two critical facts that we aren't learning from our physicians:

1. Most of us naturally begin the aging process with a loss of the hormone testosterone after age 40.
2. This condition is easily treatable.

When it is recognized, the course of the condition is progressive and symptoms parallel the drop of testosterone. Fatigue and many other symptoms appear that lead to feeling "old." Later, if testosterone is not replaced, the symptoms progress into diseases such as chronic fatigue, fibromyalgia, heart disease, stroke, memory loss, dementia, and autoimmune disorders such as rheumatoid arthritis or lupus. Many older women who do not undergo hormone therapy needlessly end up using walkers and wheelchairs. Eventually, their condition progresses to a point where they are bedridden and in nursing homes because they have lost muscle mass.

Unfortunately, because physicians think of the early signs of TDS as merely unrelated symptoms of aging, most do not recognize what is really happening. No governing body of doctors has identified these symptoms as a *specific condition* and given it a name. It has been the "secret" female syndrome for far too long!

It is time to change that.

Why Women Suffer from TDS in the First Place

Kathy's patients naturally want to know why TDS occurs and why they are experiencing the symptoms of "aging" when they have only lived half of their lives.

The explanation for the cause of TDS is likelier to be found in anthropology and human history than in medicine. There are a few excellent popular books that explain why we enter the nonre-productive phase of our lives at around age 40. I recommend two in particular: *Why Women Have Sex* by Cindy M. Meston and David M. Buss, PhDs, and *The Science of Orgasm,* by Barry R. Komisaruk, Carlos Beyer-Flores, and Beverly Whipple, PhDs.

The short answer to the question is that our life expectancy has been increasing since prehistory, from an average life span of less than 35 years to one of more than 75 today. Up until about 200 years ago, women often died in childbirth. Both sexes had shortened life spans because of lack of clean water, vaccines, and advances in medicine. Women rarely experienced TDS simply because they rarely lived long enough to reach the age of its onset; their natural life expectancy was limited to the age of reproduction. So when the loss of testosterone decreases desire and progesterone, it also causes the increased chance of miscarriage, starting about age 40.

As women's life spans have extended beyond the time they can reproduce, the age of marriage and the end of adolescence have been delayed. Unfortunately, though, the original anatom-ical equipment and hormonal "clock" have not evolved. Women still experience the loss of testosterone at the same age they did 50,000 years ago. Now that they live many years beyond fertility, they experience symptoms related to testosterone deficiency long before their lives are over. To put it simply, women now outlive their testosterone production!

This is a quality-of-life issue for women as well as a health risk. In the 21st century, living means far more than just surviving. Quality of life is the ingredient we must regain to be productive and independent as we live into our 70s, 80s, and 90s.

How We Got Here

As long as governing medical organizations do not recognize or name a condition, the group of symptoms attributed to it does not qualify for research or insurance coverage. In short, if organizations such as the FDA, the AMA, and the NIH do not acknowledge a disease, and if there is no official billing code for the problem in the government's book of diseases (known as ICD-9 codes), no one will research it, treat it, or pay to treat it!

Furthermore, successful treatment depends upon a correct diagnosis. Doctors must know the symptoms of a disease before they can diagnose and treat it appropriately. Happily, medicine has advanced to the point where once we identify a condition we can usually find a treatment. While research has been done on women and testosterone, it has focused on singular symptoms and their relationships to testosterone. I have not found any research that has put all the symptoms together to correctly describe the syndrome that affects the majority of women after age 40.

Gender Bias on the Part of the FDA and the Medical Establishment

By not recognizing or naming this syndrome that affects women, the medical establishment is continuing its history of putting women behind men in its goals for health care, research, and the development of new drugs.

But why? Isn't that era over?

Unfortunately, it isn't . . . at least not in the medical community, because top management in the government, medical societies, the research industry, and pharmaceutical companies is still male dominated. And no one has yet gotten these medical groups to look at hormone imbalances from a female perspective. Because testosterone has always been thought of as a male hormone, women have never been the primary focus of medical studies concerning it.

Mainstream medicine is still living with the belief that women and men are created completely differently. In reality, the sexes have almost all of the same organs and hormones, but we develop differently depending on the concentration of testosterone, which is present in both. In fact, men produce estrogen and women produce testosterone. Despite all of this, it is still considered a fact that women do not have (or need) testosterone. We are only now beginning to concentrate on the importance of this hormone in women.

Testosterone is not just important to women's hormonal balance, it is essential. In fact, it is our primary sex hormone, three times as abundant as estradiol throughout our lives. As you can see in the chart that follows, testosterone is actually our most abundant sex hormone. Why aren't we told that?

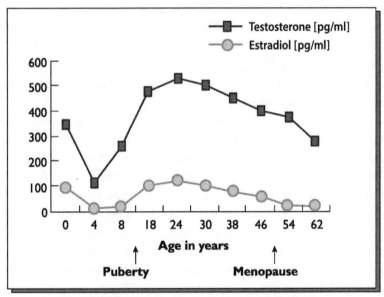

The blood level of testosterone is always three times as high as estradiol in women throughout reproductive life.

Because of the gender dynamics cited earlier, it is easier to approve drugs for men than for women, and drugs primarily for men have more rapid approval processes. Let us compare the erectile dysfunction (ED) drug Viagra and the testosterone patch for women. Both drugs are for sexual functioning, yet the FDA approved Viagra in just six months after only three studies had been conducted. Compared to the rest of the drugs that are approved for use, this is very fast! In contrast, the female testosterone patch was scrutinized for years with three to four times as many studies, and then it was prevented from being released in the U.S. because of a concern regarding potential facial hair production as a side effect. And while facial hair is obviously not life threatening, Viagra can cause sudden death from cardiac collapse.

The FDA Won't Approve Bio-identical Testosterone for Women

Bio-identical testosterone is the most effective form of treatment with the least risk for both men and women. It is plant based, created by a special pharmacy that makes it from yams and soy. It is not produced by a big pharmaceutical company and can be made in any dose for which a doctor writes a prescription on behalf of an individual patient.

FDA approvals of testosterone differ for men and women. For men who have "andropause" (low testosterone production), also called hypogonadism, bio-identical testosterone in pellet form— the form I believe to be by far the most effective—is one of several FDA-approved types of testosterone replacement. For women suffering from low testosterone levels, the story is quite different: Estratest, an oral combination of methyltestosterone and estrogen, is unfortunately the only FDA-approved testosterone.

Bio-identical hormones such as testosterone are not FDA approved for women in *any* form, including the pellet form approved for men. Yet bio-identical pellets are extremely safe and effective. They are a legal and economical "off-label" use for women in the treatment of testosterone deficiency. Later on, you'll learn more about what "off-label" use means.

Unfortunately, bio-identical pellets are just not as widely available as they would be if they were FDA approved for this purpose.

Testosterone Has an Unearned Bad Reputation

When we think of testosterone, we often picture someone who takes it transforming into the Hulk, with bulging muscles and a bad temperament. We'll say, "That guy has too much testosterone," when a man irrationally overreacts, commits a violent act, or is too macho. This is simply an unearned assumption that has worked its way into our vernacular.

When Kathy was a resident in OB/GYN, there was only one other woman in the residency with her; in the early 1980s women were not welcomed into the male-dominated world of OB/GYN. Once at a department meeting, she felt there were a lot of problems with equality that were preventing people from doing their jobs, so she spoke up. She knew there would be more women to come after her and that these problems should be rectified to make the path easier, even if speaking up made hers harder. As she walked out of the meeting, a member of the department who has since become its chief asked her if he could look under her skirt to see if she had balls, because she obviously had too much testosterone! Today, that may seem unbelievable, but at that time testosterone in women was negatively associated with assertiveness!

To make matters worse, the misuse of anabolic steroids caused medical testosterone to be associated with illegal use. Testosterone has been in medical use for more than three quarters of a century, since the early 1930s, and has never been illegal when prescribed by a doctor. Not only is it legal when administered in synthetic and bio-identical forms by a licensed physician for certain approved conditions in men; it is an *essential* hormone that should be replaced in both women and men who suffer from hormone deficiency.

UNDERSTANDING THE TERMINOLOGY: "LEGAL," "REGULATED," AND "APPROVED"

To understand the allegations against testosterone, it is helpful to be aware of the terms that differentiate classes of drugs.

Testosterone is a controlled substance. That means that the DEA monitors the distribution and use of this hormone as if it were a narcotic, even though it isn't. It is not habit forming like other controlled drugs, but it has been misused in the past by young athletes, so it is watched by regulatory agencies in the United States.

The two federal agencies that are involved in the regulatory process for drug manufacturing and distribution in the United States are the DEA and the FDA. The DEA is the watching agency and classifies testosterone as *legal* under appropriate medical conditions. It *regulates* testosterone in every form in the U.S., like other "habit-forming" or "dangerous" prescription drugs. Of course, testosterone is classified as addictive and dangerous, but when used appropriately under a physician's supervision, it is neither of those things. The DEA is worried about abuse and misuse by athletes and young teens, so it regulates it as a schedule III drug.

The FDA regulates the production and manufacturing of all drugs made by pharmaceutical companies and gives patients the following four assurances:

1. The product is pure.
2. The dose on the label is consistent with the drug.
3. It is dispensed in a way that leaves a paper trail.
4. There are lot numbers and expiration dates on the drug in case there is a recall.

For compounded bio-identical hormones made by a compounding pharmacy, the states' Bureau of Narcotics and Dangerous Drugs (BNDD) provides this assurance state by state. If there is a violation, then the FDA comes in to rectify the problem. Luckily, this has rarely happened. These regulations are considered a protection for patients, because a patient who receives a legally dispensed, regulated drug like testosterone is guaranteed to receive the drug in pure form and assured that it will always be the same dose within a small percentage variance.

The term "approved by the FDA" is different from "regulated by the FDA" or BNDD. Approval represents yet another level of restriction beyond regulation. When the FDA approves, or sanctions, drugs, it officially authorizes their use for a particular diagnosis or set of diagnoses, and *only* to treat a specific illness or disease. This, however, does *not* restrict doctors from using a drug for other diseases or symptoms, beyond those approved parameters.

Many people mistakenly assume that if a drug is not approved, it is not legal and not available. They do not realize that not only is it *legal* to use a drug in a nonapproved fashion, but it happens all the time and often with terrific results. This is done across the medical profession by mainstream physicians in almost every discipline. It is well recognized among doctors that many drugs that are tested for safety, dosage, and effectiveness by the FDA for one disease are in fact very effective for an entirely different disease. When doctors use these drugs in ways that are not approved by the FDA, it is referred to as an off-label use.

Off-Label Use

There are of course ramifications to off-label use. For instance, malpractice liability insurance companies may not cover a drug that is used outside of the purpose for which it is approved. In this case, doctors who decide to use a drug for nonapproved purposes may risk voiding their insurance if something were to go wrong. However, malpractice insurance can be amended to accommodate this practice.

Many physicians are quite aware that a drug is not approved for a certain purpose, yet regularly and routinely use it for that purpose anyway. There are many examples of physicians using drugs "off label" long before the FDA approved them for a second diagnosis. Following are a few of them:

- Topamax was approved as an antiseizure medication in 1996, but physicians recognized it as a miracle drug that could prevent migraine headaches and regularly prescribed it for prevention and treatment of migraines for many years before the FDA approved it for this purpose in 2004.

- Terbutaline is the generic name for an FDA-approved asthma drug produced and prescribed for this purpose in the 1970s. During this time, it was used off label in labor and delivery as the first-line drug for premature labor, although it was never approved for any other diagnosis than asthma.

- Spironolactone (brand name Aldactone) was originally approved for the treatment of high blood pressure and as a water pill. It was a very weak diuretic, but doctors soon discovered it was much more effective as a preventive measure for facial hair growth and acne in women and used it regularly for these purposes, for which it has never been approved.

We could list many other drugs that have been researched and developed by pharmaceutical companies for one disease and then prescribed by creative physicians for other diseases, when there is no effective approved medication. Physicians are very inventive when they need a treatment for their patients. Still, some very conservative physicians take a narrow view of off-label uses of medications and their patients miss out on the use of excellent drugs. Despite a medication's ability to treat a disease other than the one for which it has been approved, these physicians view the FDA's stamp of approval as the last word in deciding whether or not to prescribe a drug, regardless of how much a patient may benefit from the off-label drug.

Lack of Funding Impacts FDA Approval

Why doesn't the FDA extend approvals for the use of off-label drugs like testosterone, when physicians have recognized they are useful for other purposes?

The answer is money. It takes many millions of dollars in testing and research to get a drug approved for a particular diagnosis. When a medication becomes generic, it is not patentable or exclusively "own-able" by any pharmaceutical company, and as a result there is no opportunity for profit. It is therefore not cost effective for a company to pay the considerable expense of research on a second use of the drug or the use on a different population of patients. If there is no pharmaceutical company championing a drug for a certain disease, it is unlikely the FDA will approve it for that purpose, regardless of its proven effectiveness!

IF GYNECOLOGISTS DON'T KNOW ABOUT TDS, WHO DOES?

There are very few articles dedicated to hormones in the OB/GYN literature. Most in the major journals are centered on the complexities of fertility and pregnancy, not pre- or postmenopause. Since OB/GYNs often act as women's primary-care physicians, this creates a major problem for women when they start to encounter symptoms of testosterone loss.

If gynecologists don't read about the research on testosterone replacement in the journals published by their specialty, where can they find it? Endocrinology is a medical specialty that branches from internal medicine, not gynecology, and researches both men and women. Its journals are where most of the research on female menopause, hormone imbalance, and testosterone deficiency can be found. Yet endocrinologists generally do not treat women with menopause or other female hormone disorders because that is clinically an OB/GYN's job. Thus there is a giant chasm between the treating physician and the research being done on testosterone for women!

In other words, hormone replacement therapy currently has no designated place in the medical world. Therefore, there are no medical professionals in any specialty who see women for hormone deficiencies and are adequately trained to identify and treat the group of symptoms associated with hormone loss in mature women. The consequence is that OB/GYNs just dismiss it as the normal aging process and return their focus to their pregnant patients. On the other hand, endocrinologists read the literature but aren't trained and do not engage in the practice of treating women's hormones.

Enter the specialty of antiaging medicine, which treats both women and men with deficient hormones.

It's Time for a Middle-aged Women's Medical Bill of Rights

Women over 40 have enough life experience to realize that they have been left behind by the medical system. Those "of a certain age" participated in the battles for Title IX and other protections for women in the 1970s. Today women have the right to be listened to—not dismissed as "hormonal" or "old" and therefore irrelevant. Women deserve to be heard and taken seriously on this issue. It is time these symptoms no longer are considered the result of the normal aging process, but an eminently treatable condition called testosterone deficiency syndrome, or TDS. And it's time our need for treatment is met.

Everyone deserves a valid explanation for pain and other changes in their bodies that take them by surprise at midlife.

Ask Your Doctor: A Summary

Armed with the information in this chapter, when you notice signs of TDS, you can discuss the option of hormone replacement therapy and have the data to approach your doctor on a more equal footing. You can understand their reason for using or not using testosterone or other bio-identicals, and you can find a physician who can objectively discuss this safe, legal, and effective option with you.

Fortunately, this can now happen easily and affordably. There is a cure for the symptoms that kill our productivity and steal our happiness, and it is just a pellet away.

CHAPTER 3

How TDS Triggers the Aging Cascade

Every woman starts the aging cascade at around 40 years of age when she begins the transition from the reproductive to the postreproductive stage of her life. The aging cascade is simply the sequential loss of three hormones, one after the other. Testosterone is the first to go, then progesterone, then estradiol. We have identified the symptoms relating to the first stage of aging as TDS. Let's now look at this process as a whole.

Progression of Hormone Loss after Age 40

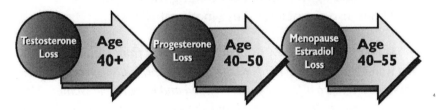

TESTOSTERONE: THE FIRST HORMONE TO FALL

At 39, Ellen had a "perfect" body, and she worked hard to maintain it. She ate well and exercised, drank lots of water, and rarely drank alcohol. In fact, she loved to exercise and ran five to ten miles every other day. On the nonrunning days, she lifted weights or did Pilates. All of her friends were in awe of her beautiful body . . . then she hit 40. Her waistline started to expand, so she ate less. She tried every diet and exercised more. Her hair started to fall out, she lost the color in her face, and she looked tired and older than her years. By the time she sought help, her spirit was broken. She had been a superwoman; intense training and exercise had never failed her before. She wanted to know what was wrong so she could fix it!

Testosterone deficiency begins by adversely affecting physical appearance. Around the age of 40, women see their bodies begin to change and age. Their breasts are no longer perky, their waistlines disappear, their muscles are no longer toned, and their facial features start to sag.

None of us wants to be considered vain, but what does a woman do when she suddenly feels as though she is living in someone else's body? Like Ellen, they try diets and exercise programs to no avail and end up feeling as though they have no control over their own bodies. The reality is that they simply cannot control their weight, waistline, and figure without controlling their hormones.

TDS is also characterized by emotional changes.

When Kerri turned 47, she looked at pictures from her 20s and 30s and wondered what had happened to that vibrant, smiling person. These days, she felt like a different person—a sad and haggard old woman. Her sadness showed all over her face and she worried that she would never be the same. When she polled her friends, they confided that they were feeling the same way! They all wondered, What happened?!

The fact that women's looks change is not generally what makes them depressed; they expect *some* change as they age. But the mood changes are unexpected. Usually, "moodiness" or "funk" is treated with antidepressants. These drugs provide an increase in the neuro-hormone serotonin instead of homing in on the true cause: the depleted sex hormone testosterone.

Vigor for life, sexual desire and responsiveness, motivation to participate, calm in a storm, and mood stability often disappear. Women become irritable, they wonder where this all came from, and none of the experts they seek for answers do anything more than put the Band-Aid of drugs over this emotional cataclysm. The result is a loss of self-esteem that negatively impacts their relationships and families.

Why Do We Have Chemical Imbalances?

Anxiety and depression are common, and they are difficult to treat because even though we understand the chemical imbalance that causes them, we do not understand the original cause of the imbalance—the first thing that used up or suppressed the chemicals in our brain and started the ball rolling. Treatment traditionally includes counseling sessions that help us develop strategies for functioning in life with these disabilities and medications that will make the journey easier.

Antidepressants are often given to treat mood disorders created by low testosterone. Yet, paradoxically, as part of their function, they suppress the production of testosterone, thereby compounding the sexual problem by lowering libido and responsiveness. End result: you have to choose between being less depressed or maintaining your sex drive. Of course, depression itself often reduces the sex drive. The choice becomes this: do we want to have a stable mood, or do we want to sustain our love relationships?

The discovery of TDS changes this for women who develop anxiety and depression after age 38 and helps us understand the role testosterone plays in both depression and anxiety. Not only is low testosterone a concrete causative factor, but it is measurable and curable.

PROGESTERONE: THE SECOND HORMONE TO FALL

Unpredictable progesterone production begins when women are in their 40s and early 50s and the ovaries stop regularly ovulating, which eliminates progesterone production on a month-by-month basis. This causes a periodic loss of progesterone and increased production of estradiol, the estrogen made by young women. As women age and go through menopause, they make less estradiol and begin to make estrone, another form of estrogen.

The second step of the aging cascade is the loss of progesterone. This is often called "estrogen dominance" or "unopposed" estrogen; the loss of progesterone means there is nothing to balance estrogen. The loss of progesterone as a result of inadequate or absent ovulation is the trigger that causes this imbalance in ovarian hormones.

Symptoms of inadequate progesterone include irregular periods and heavy bleeding, PMS, breast enlargement and tenderness, bloating, swelling, poor sleep, and mood swings. These symptoms can occur at any age; however, PMS occurs universally among women after testosterone production falls. Younger women often have hormone imbalances as well, but these are generally less frequent. PMS is normally thought of as an emotional issue and not a hormone imbalance, so there is a negative connotation related to this label. Women who suffer from PMS and its symptoms are often given psychiatric drugs instead of progesterone. The most direct treatment in all age groups is to replace the missing progesterone, and in women over 40, progesterone and testosterone are given for complete resolution. Many women could be saved the expense of psychiatric drugs, antidepressants, and antianxiety drugs to treat PMS—and avoid the side effects that come with these drugs—simply by replacing the missing progesterone their bodies used to make!

ESTRADIOL: THE THIRD HORMONE TO FALL

Estradiol is the third and final hormone we lose in the aging cascade and everything that comes with feeling old. This loss triggers symptoms of menopause such as dry vagina, painful intercourse, lack of periods, recurrent urinary tract infections, anxiety, poor sleep, and the ever-popular "hot flashes." Most women know more about menopause than any other stage of aging, but what they aren't aware of is how the loss of this hormone and those before it trigger all of the symptoms of aging they consider inevitable. Because these deficiencies occur in midlife and significantly impair the second half of life, it is important to at least consider halting this process. These hormones are easily replaced, with very low risk and very high return.

All the hormone decreases in the aging process, including the progressive loss of growth hormone (GH), stem from the pituitary gland. Initially GH decreases in response to the initial loss of testosterone and continues to fall throughout the process of estradiol and progesterone loss. We will discuss GH in detail in the following chapters as a companion hormone that parallels testosterone.

Remember: even young women may have these symptoms if they have experienced the following circumstances:

- Adrenal failure (Addison's disease) or removal
- Head injury
- Low thyroid hormone
- Lupron therapy for endometriosis
- Pituitary tumor or injury
- Premature menopause
- Removal of the ovaries
- Stroke
- Use of birth control pills

Now that we've looked at the aging cascade and the loss of testosterone, progesterone, and estradiol, we can take a closer look at the impact of testosterone loss. But before we do so, we want to talk about the importance of sex and libido in our lives in general. We are a curious mix of physical and cultural beings; we interpret and label much of what we experience physically from a cultural perspective. For example, when children are young and learning to eat "grown-up" food, they are instructed by their parents about how to interpret the sensations involved. If a child is given spicy foods and all the surrounding cultural information is that these are good feelings and good tastes, the child learns to recognize that hot (spicy) foods are a delicacy and are good things to eat. If that child were given the same foods as a punishment for being "bad," he or she would associate the sensations of spicy food with something negative and undesirable. To carry this analogy further, we also learn cultural messages about attractiveness. How we dress, wear our hair, and use makeup and even our body shape are all encapsulated in cultural messages we receive through the media and from our families.

The same is true of sexual things. There are cultural messages about what is desirable, appropriate, dirty, and shameful that we receive from our culture, our family, and our religion. For example, as a therapist, Brett has worked with many women who were taught that girls do not masturbate. It is something shameful and sinful, and no self-respecting and decent lady does that. Obviously many women no longer are limited by this cultural message, and the world is changing with regard to this behavior and its acceptance.

What we feel sexually from our physical arousal is organic. How we interpret and use it is relational and cultural. When our bodies change and the physical sensations diminish or disappear, this reality impacts the way we experience ourselves and the way others experience us. For this reason, we have included the first chapter of Part II, which gives us an opportunity to take a look at sex and libido.

A DEEPER LOOK AT THE CRITICAL HORMONES

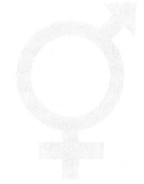

CHAPTER 4

SEX AND TESTOSTERONE

"He just wanted to have sex once a month, but I couldn't even do that! I know it is terrible of me, but I just hate it when he touches me!"

Prior to turning 40, Wendy had a higher-than-average sex drive and had once enjoyed a very satisfying sex life with her husband. After 40, she felt betrayed by her own body.

"I don't know what's wrong with me! I pick on him on nights when we usually have sex just so I don't have to do it! I love him, but I don't want to have sex anymore. What's wrong with me?"

Wendy, like so many women her age, found her lack of sexual desire beginning to erode her relationship with her husband, Doug. Wendy said he was hurt and confused. Doug said, "Sex is important to me and was a very important part of our marriage for the last 20 years. Then one day I came home and she told me she's done with this part of her life. It's over and she's not having sex anymore! I couldn't believe it! Bait and switch, that's what it was. Have great sex for the first part of the marriage, and then just unilaterally decide it is over. I'm not going to be able to do this for the rest of my life!"

In this chapter we look closely at the issues of aging and how loss of libido impacts our lives. This happens to all of us as we age. Over time, we lose the amount of testosterone our bodies made when we were young, and this occurs regardless of whether we are in a relationship or not. Even those of us who have celibate lifestyles will feel changes in our level of desire and in our ability to deny ourselves sexual satisfaction. Arousal and desire are original-issue equipment, and this portion of our equipment comes on line when we hit puberty. As we age, our equipment begins to deteriorate; we feel less arousal and less desire.

What happens to a relationship when the sex drive dies for one of the partners but not the other? A tremendous challenge to the survival and maintenance of the relationship arises when partners no longer cuddle, nurture physically, or have sex, and lose that avenue of intimacy.

THE EPIDEMIC OF SEXLESSNESS

Sex is great. It helps us feel good physically, and it helps us feel good about who we are and how loved we are. Couples who have a healthy sex life live longer and report more satisfaction in their lives than those who do not. Is that really a surprise? Probably not. And yet, sexlessness among those over 40 is on the rise these days. This is the subject of discussion everywhere from *Oprah* and *Dr. Phil* to numerous books climbing the bestseller charts. In *The Sex-Starved Marriage*, Michele Weiner Davis explains that "only 40 percent of married couples say they're very satisfied with their sex lives." *New York* magazine wrote a recent story called "Generation Sexless"—about young New Yorkers so busy with their careers and demanding toddlers that they have little time or desire for sex. Al Cooper of the San Jose Marital and Sexuality Center says that diminished sex drive is such a problem today that it's considered the "common cold of sexual issues of the new millennium."

The big issue is that a sexless relationship is rarely a joint decision and more often a one-sided loss of libido in one partner. Anyone can lose their libido and for any number of reasons. But most often it is the woman, and it usually occurs around the age of 40 as a result of TDS. This loss is so subtle that at first we might think the change we're feeling is caused by something else, usually a hectic lifestyle that has taken away our desire. We write it off as fatigue from the care of our children, work-related stress, or even conflict with our spouse. Pretty soon, we "forget" about feeling sexy and stop responding to flirting and sexual advances. When our partner tries to initiate sex, we don't pick up on the signal. We are too busy; the bills need to be paid, the grass needs to be cut, the laundry needs to be done, there is a meeting at church, and the kids need to do homework. Sex is just one more thing on our never-ending to-do list.

Along with loss of libido, other symptoms of TDS are kicking in: women experience weight gain from abdominal fat, hair loss, sagging breasts, chin hair, poor skin tone, and cellulite. As you might suspect, this leads many women to feel unattractive, and they don't want to be touched or want any additional "demands" from their partner. They lose the energy for flirting and the confidence and motivation to be sexy. Understandably, the confusion and frustration they often feel with themselves translates into irritability, which makes them difficult to live with.

The husband, still possessing a healthy libido until at least the age of 55, invariably becomes acutely conscious that his wife no longer desires him. He sneaks up on ways to softly and subtly inquire: "Is it me?" "Is there something wrong?" "Are you mad?" or "Do you feel bad?" He makes these assumptions because the pattern has changed, and he does not know how to understand it. Perhaps if he knew it was a chemical change, he would have more compassion for the situation.

His partner initially answers with surprised negatives: "Not now—you just don't understand. Of course I love you and want you. It's just that I'm not in the mood. Give me a little time. I'm just distracted." Time passes, and the questions become more intense. The "Why not?" becomes louder. Often the partner who desires more sex becomes sarcastic, passive-aggressive, manipulative, seductive, and angry. The vicious cycle starts. The husband feels like he has been the victim of a bait and switch, and the wife, not feeling the same drive and feeling angry that her husband would consider sex so important, becomes even more defensive and avoidant.

Self-Esteem, Sexiness, and Libido

In our culture, sex is one of the most interesting parts of conversations. It is in every TV show and almost every advertisement. Even the thought of it is motivating and energizing for many people. When you have the right amount of active testosterone, you can engage in this subconscious dance: making yourself attractive, getting your hair and nails done, wearing that little black dress that every woman has, pampering yourself, and radiating "come hither" to the world. You know you have "it" and you want to flaunt it. When that part of a woman's personality fades, however, it can be devastating to her self-esteem.

"I am a terrible flirt, or at least I used to be," Kathy's patient Jenny reported. "For as long as I could remember, I could silence a room when I walked in with how I looked and that invisible sexuality that was always with me. I had confidence that I would get attention from the opposite sex. Then it all changed! I felt like I had a brain and body transplant. I had anxiety attacks about going to parties and gatherings. My ability to attract and chat up guys left. I didn't do anything different, but I was abandoned by my own sexuality and confidence."

Some women transition into this loss of libido without a feeling of "altered self," but to most, like Jenny, the loss of libido feels like a personality change, a loss of oneself. The loss of sexuality can be as devastating as the loss of memory, compassion, or any other character trait. Without sexuality many women find themselves adrift, alienated from their culture, their partner, and even themselves. Their entire view of the world and how they act in it can change. Remember that identifying as a girl or boy starts when we are toddlers!

When Kathy's beautiful toddler went to nursery school, she knew very well that her mom was a doctor. Kathy picked her up one afternoon and she declared, "Mom, you shouldn't be a doctor. Boys are doctors. You should be a nurse!" Such are the gender roles that we ingrain in our children so early in life. To have your gender identity—as a beautiful, sexually vibrant, and healthy woman—ripped from you in midlife is devastating.

When people lose their sexuality, they may lose their confidence in interpersonal skills and feel that others respond to them differently. Self-esteem is replaced by self-doubt and depression. For a marriage or a long-term-partner relationship, the loss of libido is so devastating it can almost be like suffering a stroke because, like a stroke, the loss of testosterone and libido is a silent killer of our basic personality.

THE ROLE OF WOMEN'S SEXUALITY IN OUR CULTURE IS CHANGING BECAUSE THEY LIVE LONGER

All mammals—and humans are mammals—are built to reproduce, and no matter how sophisticated we become as a society, women's bodies are still dedicated to that purpose. Their sex hormones' primary function is to promote fertility on a monthly basis, as long as they are healthy and young. Like all other mammals, they have a life expectancy that is limited by their reproductive time frame. Interestingly, we humans have improved our health enough to become the only mammals that outlive our reproductive years. An average woman's window of fertility occurs between the ages of 12 and 40, while her life expectancy far exceeds that. No matter how hard medicine has worked, women's lives have been prolonged but not their years of fertility. Eventually, their ovaries stop making testosterone, progesterone, and estrogen.

Why does this happen? After 40, fertility becomes an unnecessary use of energy, so testosterone drops to decrease a woman's desire to have sex. That way, she can conserve her energy to care for the children she already has. This is the same as it was in antiquity. This process allows time for the children to grow and become somewhat independent before the death of their mothers, which was meant to happen when menopause occurred.

Now women are outliving their testosterone, libido, and fertility. But for many women, the facts about the *timing* of their loss of libido and *the hormone responsible* for that change have eluded medical researchers and mainstream medicine. The professional literature on libido on which physicians rely is problematic because most of it begins with the premise that loss of libido is the result of the lack of estrogen after women's periods stop.

The fact is that the problem is TDS—loss of testosterone, not menopause. TDS is the first step in aging and the end of the female sex drive, and it occurs as much as ten years *before* menopause. After ten years of testosterone loss, women finally enter menopause when they are depleted of estrogen and eggs. This is the final stage of their childbearing capabilities, not the first.

For women, the loss of sex drive and sexual activity after 40 creates not only a great void but also an impediment to their health and happiness. Women are sexual beings; throughout their lives sex is one of their greatest pleasures. In the 21st century, when they may live to 90 or 100, should they be expected to live without sex? Should they lose the desires, the fantasies, and the emotional bonding that occur in sexually active relationships for more than 50 years?

Libido and Testosterone in Youth

To fully understand our current social problem stemming from the loss of the sex drive in middle-aged women, it is important to understand, first, *why* libido is hardwired into our brains, and second, *how* libido plays a part in our lives in the first 40 years. Because libido is testosterone dependent, testosterone is where it all begins.

When testosterone production kicks in at puberty, or even before girls start having periods, it sends the sex drive soaring. This should not be a surprise to anyone who has lived through the teenage years, when sex often dominates a person's thoughts. As we all know, the drive to think about and have sex can be nearly unstoppable during this period of life.

Significant testosterone production continues after our teenage years and into our 30s. It then plateaus for a few years before starting to disappear around the age of 40, taking the libido with it. In other words, the increase and decrease of libido in women's bodies simply parallel the levels of testosterone in their systems.

Sexual desire is just as normal as hunger and the need for sleep. And testosterone is the power source for a woman's built-in sexual drive. This drive is critical because it motivates women to have sex and become pregnant, a phenomenon that is vital to the survival of the human race. These are the basic drives and biology our ancestors have experienced from the beginning of time. We can't change our basic human nature.

An Age-Old Dance

Lack of testosterone was an obvious marker of lack of fertility in the early stages of human history.

Picture the caveman on one side of the river, viewing a cavewoman on the other side. He has to determine whether it is worth it to swim across the river to have sex. It was probably as basic as that.

Two visible signs of fertility are breasts and a small waist. (This is why breast implants and tummy tucks are so popular even today.) When the caveman looks over and sees a woman without a waistline, he determines she is either pregnant (meaning he cannot fulfill his purpose), old (the lack of testosterone increases estrone, which causes increased belly fat), or sick. He opts for staying on his side of the river to find someone with a waistline, an indication of a woman who might be more able to produce an offspring!

When Testosterone Decreases, Estrone Increases

T =Testosterone E_I =Estrone

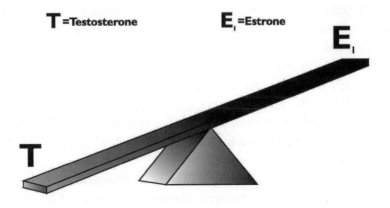

Women possess a relationship between testosterone, which is made in the ovary, and estrone, which is produced by the adrenal gland. When we are young, testosterone suppresses estrone; and as we age, low levels of testosterone allow estrone to increase.

Why Didn't My Grandmother Experience This Problem?

Before we address the fairly simple solution to this critical problem, we should first answer the question so many of my patients ask me: why is loss of libido an issue for our generation when it did not seem to be for our mothers' generation?

First, no generation is the same as the last. The world our mothers lived in was very different from ours, and that changes everything!

The generations born prior to 1945 considered sex to be a very private issue, between husband and wife. Many women were virgins when they got married, mostly because of the fear of pregnancy, which was taboo outside of marriage. Our mothers accepted their marital sex life and had nothing to compare it to.

When their libido waned after 40, they assumed that was normal, too. They also did not expect to live past 65, so at 40 they felt like they were in the last part of their lives and considered it the normal and logical course of events. Given all this conditioning, it is no surprise that our forebears did not complain about a lack of libido. In fact, they never talked about sex. If they were not interested in their husbands anymore, they turned them away or participated in body only. They were very different from today's 40-year-old woman.

These same women, who are now in their late 60s, early 70s, and older, were expected to be *generally* less assertive than we are in the 21st century, and they were habituated to the male-oriented society that defined America. Because of this, they often continued to have sex long after their desire evaporated. They considered it their duty.

Those of us born after 1945, the baby boomers, have higher expectations than our parents and grandparents did. Also, we are a much more rebellious group, and far less ready to accept any particular status quo. In other words, women boomers are not as inclined to accept a male-dominated society as were their mothers and grandmothers.

We could say that the Age of Aquarius spawned an entirely new kind of woman. With the advent of birth control, women who grew up in the 1960s and 1970s had a newfound freedom and became much more open about sex, both in word and deed. At hundreds of flower-power concerts, they gave their libidos free rein and partook in the "free love" that was a hallmark of the era. This was the first generation in thousands of years to bring sex out into the open and acknowledge that women enjoy sex as much as men. This new way of thinking gave women a fuller life and an unprecedented sexual equality with men.

Over time, however, the sexual revolution of the '60s and '70s proved to be a mixed blessing for this pioneering generation of women because their expectations set them up for a major disappointment. They had embraced their sexuality while their mothers had buried theirs, yet it never occurred to them that their sex drive would disappear. Since the cause of this loss is physical and not societal, they were, and are, greatly disappointed. Expecting to live and have sex forever, they felt a catastrophic loss that their grandmothers and mothers did not experience when their libidos disappeared with their testosterone.

Many of these women feel this loss more acutely and feel more incomplete in their 40s than their mothers did. Their mothers did not expect to be sexually active past 40. Moreover, no one warned our generation about this change. For many of us, it was like losing our sight; once we have had it, we experience its loss even more severely!

Many of the songs of the '60s and '70s were about living forever and never accepting the status quo. That spirit traveled with women as they aged, even if their testosterone did not. Many women in this age group express this feeling of being tricked by their own bodies when they lament the loss of their youth and their sexual personalities; but accepting this situation—losing interest in sex as they age and quietly suffering—is not an option for them in the same way it was for their mothers. This is not a future they accept.

Although the cultural revolution of the last 50 years has freed women from many social restrictions, they are still bound by the same physiological limitations. They are smarter and healthier, and they live longer, yet they must still live with the unchanged fact that their ability to reproduce is finite and ends when their testosterone runs out in their 40s.

Here's the good news: information about how to correct these sexual losses is available, and the single answer is *testosterone*. Also, the number of women working as professionals in medicine has sky-rocketed, bringing additional revelations to light and opportunities for reclaiming women's sexuality. Researchers like Beverly Whipple, RN, PhD, who solved the mystery of orgasms in her book *The Science of Orgasm,* have led the charge in understanding our bodies fully. In this book, we build on that understanding and explain how we can solve the problem of libido loss triggered by TDS.

WHY MAINSTREAM MEDICINE FAILS TO DIAGNOSE AND TREAT LOW LIBIDO IN WOMEN

Mainstream medicine fails miserably in both diagnosing and treating TDS-induced loss of libido. Loss of libido is not just a symptom of aging but the most universal symptom of testosterone deprivation. Testosterone, therefore, is the single hormone women must replace to regain their sexual selves. Happily, the return of libido is the first sign that testosterone replacement is working, but unfortunately, medicine has thus far refused to acknowledge this fact. It does not recognize that testosterone impacts women in exactly the same way it does men in terms of sexuality. It stimulates desire, augments sexual performance, facilitates orgasms, and keeps the brain aware of sexual touch and invitation at all times.

Tragically, conventional medical wisdom ignores the importance of the sex drive in women and does not find it worthy of a doctor's time. Until recently, mainstream medicine espoused the notion that women didn't and shouldn't even have a sex drive. The studies state over and over again that if a woman is stimulated in a "certain way," she will respond, whether she has testosterone or not.

Traditionally, our medical world has been one of male-dominated instruction. The time has come for the medical establishment to stop dismissing women as nonsexual beings and to spend more time, energy, and money on addressing the cause of women's loss of libido. Then there might actually be true advancement in the cause of women's health.

Why is there this double standard in medical care between treating loss of libido in men and women? Sadly, women, libido, and testosterone are low on the priority list of both federal agencies and drug companies, for several reasons. First, men are the primary interest of drug companies and the FDA because, with no periods or pregnancies to worry about, they are easier to study. Second, researchers are primarily men, so they relate to the problems of men and dismiss women as unworthy subjects for scientific research. Finally, to develop a treatment standard for a particular problem, medicine has to follow these three guidelines:

1. Recognize the symptom or disease as a medical problem. The medical establishment doesn't currently recognize this for women.

2. Have concern about what will happen to the patient if the problem isn't treated. There is generally little or no concern about women's libido in medicine today.

3. Feel comfortable talking openly with their patients about the problem. Until we train doctors to comfortably talk about sex, we will not see much progress in how doctors treat sexual problems in women.

Biologic Actions of Testosterone in Women
Activates overall brain activity and memory
Acts as an anti-inflammatory agent
Decreases risk of Alzheimer's disease and dementia
Decreases risk of cancer
Improves balance
Improves immunity
Improves insulin resistance
Improves mood and reduces anxiety
Increases blood flow to muscles
Increases bone strength—both absorption of calcium and vitamin D to increase bone growth
Increases energy
Increases growth hormone, which increases lean body mass
Increases libido
Increases muscle growth, thus decreases frailty
Increases production of both red and white cells
Increases skin thickness
Reduces cholesterol in the blood
Reduces obesity
Stabilizes brain neurotransmitters to decrease migraine headaches

THE EFFECT OF THIS DOUBLE STANDARD ON TESTOSTERONE REPLACEMENT

As we have outlined, our current societal priorities for male drugs leave research on drugs for women without necessary resources. As a result, testosterone is more than a decade behind cholesterol drugs in terms of being commonly prescribed for women. Most OB/GYNs don't even consider testosterone as a treatment because it's not a standard of care for women. As a result, there is no way to prescribe it to women except by working outside the system; therefore, most doctors do not do it. Instead, they spout the outdated bromide that estrogen is the primary female hormone. Not true! Women make three times more testosterone than estradiol when they are young and healthy.

We are also sadly lacking in research on testosterone's effects on sexuality in women. Drug companies have managed to pass through the FDA just one drug for women containing a synthetic testosterone, even though, not surprisingly, there are more than four erectile dysfunction (ED) drugs and dozens of different FDA-approved testosterone preparations for men to choose from. Urologists and internal medicine doctors are given boxes of ED drugs from drug representatives that they readily hand out to their male patients.

The single drug for women is a synthetic testosterone administered orally, Estratest. When this preparation was poorly received by women because of its side effects (increased anger and excessive facial hair—side effects that are not present with bio-identical forms of testosterone), medical "intellectuals" concluded that women just didn't need it, instead of condemning the form of testosterone that Estratest contained. This certainly hasn't happened with male preparations. When one form of testosterone for men was not adequate or had undesirable side effects, researchers quickly developed other kinds of testosterone preparations. Mainstream medical research papers denigrate all medications that are considered "testosteronelike" for women as ineffective or "risky." Is this the outcome of the parochial view of women's ability to need and enjoy sex? Or is it a disregard for the needs of women?

When women seek their doctors' help for loss of libido, their experiences are far different from men's experiences. There are no samples of testosterone medication to hand out to women. Their physicians don't have answers to the problem, so they tell women to simply live with it as a way of avoiding the problem.

Annie is a high school science teacher who calmly states that she went to four doctors before seeing a hormone specialist. Her lifelong gynecologist answered her inquiry about her lost libido at 40 by chuckling and saying that by now she should be tired of sex—why would she want to have a libido again? He told her to see a psychiatrist. She dutifully made an appointment with one, who told her that she was sane and had no psychological problems and that her lost libido must stem from depression. She was prescribed an antidepressant. Within two weeks of taking it, she was fatigued and had even less sex drive than before, so she stopped taking the pills. Then her husband suggested she see his medical doctor. After a thorough exam, he told Annie that she was just fine and that she was just getting old; she would just have to live with it. At this point, she said sadly that she really did feel depressed. An acupuncturist was her next visit in her attempt to find a cure, but to no avail. Finally, she went to see the hormone doctor whom her hairdresser had recommended. She broke down during this visit and said that if she was not cured this time, she was just going to give up. Fortunately, she finally found the answer. Annie regained her life and her marriage with the replacement of testosterone.

How Much Sex Is "Normal"?

When couples come to us, either for testosterone replacement or counseling, inevitably one of the partners wants to know what "normal" is in regard to frequency of intercourse. In reality, couples develop their own typical frequency, depending on their libidos and opportunity. For some couples, having sex daily is normal, and for others, even when they are young, having sex once a month is the norm. This negotiated "normal" is specific to them, and when that changes because of loss of libido, the partner with a normal libido is left without an outlet for their sexuality. They begin to feel that there is something wrong with their relationship or that the partner without a libido has somehow decided to "change the rules" of the relationship. This, of course, causes conflict.

To evaluate your relationship, don't go back to your first year of being a couple to consider the "normal" for you. Instead, think about the fourth or fifth year together when the rhythm of life brought your sexual activity to a baseline. Then review together the things that might have changed your frequency over the years, such as the birth of a child, a parent moving into your home, or the stress of work. After that you can arrive at a conclusion as to whether your sex life has come to a crisis because of external stress or one partner withdrawing because of loss of desire.

The best way to determine if testosterone deficiency is the problem is to first balance, or replace, both partners' hormones. Then review expectations, since our sexual satisfaction often grows from a hormone balance in both partners.

Beth, one of our patients, wrote us about her "new" life on testosterone. She and her husband were in the bathtub together on a Saturday afternoon. They had just had some "alone time," and they were sitting there together drinking a glass of wine. Beth's husband leaned back in the tub and looked at her and said, "I love Dr. Maupin."

Now here is couple who is approaching 60, and they're having this wonderful Saturday afternoon together that is only possible because testosterone was replaced. Women fear that when they're in their 40s, 50s, and 60s they're not going to have those bathtub moments anymore. When TDS is treated, however, they can get back to their old relationship.

In order to achieve this kind of result, subcutaneous bio-identical pellets are the best method. This means of providing the restoration of testosterone causes the body to once again experience the delivery of testosterone in a natural, on-demand way to support the libido and reengage all the functions of testosterone described in this book. Pellets dissolve somewhat slowly and create a stable level for three to four months, when another dose must be given. Women who replace their testosterone will know that the aging cascade has been defeated or delayed to a significant degree when they enjoy the return of their sex drive. (For more on testosterone pellets, see Chapter 9.)

Communication is critical to addressing this problem with your doctor, but communication is just as important after hormone replacement brings your hormones to pre-TDS levels. Couples must often take a chance and learn to speak their expectations out loud, in a nonconfrontational manner. The rule in this type of communication is that you have to ask for what you want in order to get it. Mind reading is rarely the optimal mode to bring back a satisfying sex life. It may take time, counseling, and communication to return to the sexual frequency and satisfaction you enjoyed as a normal, young, healthy couple.

There are often religious or cultural barriers to this type of thinking, let alone to experimentation. Couples who are working on these issues will be encouraged to take a series of low-risk steps to try to engage each other. Remember: your brain is your most sexual organ. If we can get you to think about and then verbalize even a small portion of what you want, think, or feel, you will make progress in exploring and expanding your repertoire of communication.

ASK BRETT

"I have been taking blood-pressure medicine, and now that I turned 40 I have been given an antidepressant. I find that I do not think about having sex anymore. I just don't feel sexy, and I have trouble getting turned on with my boyfriend. I love him, but something doesn't feel right. What should I do?"—Sharon, 40

Doctors often prescribe medicines in order to treat what they see as life-threatening conditions. Unfortunately, they can have side effects that impact other areas of your life—and the overall quality of life. However, there are strategies you and your boyfriend can use to overcome them.

First, you should communicate all of these emotions to your boyfriend. Doing this will help him see that your lack of responsiveness and desire isn't about him—and that will likely come as a huge relief! Explain that it is a physical issue, one that is chemically caused by the drugs you are taking. Reassure him that you still love him and *want to want* to be intimate with him. Ask your doctor about hormone replacement options and look into the possibility of bio-identical testosterone pellets as a way to ramp up your sex drive.

THE EFFECT HORMONE IMBALANCE HAS ON FAMILY RELATIONSHIPS

Months and years of hormone deprivation result in a variety of dysfunctions in marriages and ongoing relationships. Misinterpretation of the symptoms of testosterone deprivation by the partner can ultimately affect sexual relationships and significantly alter a couple's intimate milieu. Finding a way out of this desert is difficult. When we begin a relationship, so much of what we use to communicate love and desire is nonverbal, so we don't always develop a verbal sexual communication. Thus, when people attempt to reestablish their intimate relationship after treatment for TDS, or any physical illness that impairs their sexuality, they commonly find that they don't have the tools necessary to reconnect.

Sex is one of the most powerful bonding agents, so the widespread loss of testosterone, neurotransmitters, and subsequently the sexual relationship is destructive to women physically; in terms of self-esteem, sense of worth, and desirability, it is one of the most destructive forces currently threatening our monogamous culture. This loss, and the resultant loss of a sexual relationship, is one of the reasons why fully half of marriages and monogamous partnerships now fail.

This same loss of testosterone eventually happens to men, but at an older age. If men lost their desire for sex at the same age women did, the social upheaval would not be so disastrous and there would not be such a need for women to regain their slowly ebbing sex drives.

THE BIG "O"

No, I'm not talking about the magazine. Orgasm is like the weather: everyone talks about it, but few know much about it. It either happens or it does not, and no one knows why. When there are problems with orgasm, no one knows what to do to "fix" them.

We are driven to participate in sex because of the pleasure it can bring. We are made this way. We want to have sex because it is fun and feels good. And one of the most "feel-good" experiences we can have sexually is the orgasm. The brain is the most sexual organ, but it requires peripheral stimulation to get it to deliver an orgasm. A full answer requires a look at the physiology of an orgasm and the difference between orgasm and sex.

Most simply stated, adequate levels of free testosterone are fundamental to a healthy sexual drive, a healthy sex life, and orgasm. A happy relationship and even social cohesion depend on it. Unfortunately many women never experience it until they receive testosterone pellets. We have seen some of these women within a month of treatment return to our offices and announce loudly to the waiting room full of patients, "*That* is what everyone has been talking about! Thank you, thank you, thank you!"

It is a truly sad thing for a woman to go through life "anorgasmic." She feels deprived, guilty, and ashamed. These feelings are entirely unnecessarily. The principal physical cause of this condition is the lack of testosterone. If women are given an adequate amount of testosterone, they become orgasmic. Our bodies are made to work that way; when they do not, there is a reason. Obviously, anorgasmic conditions may have other causes such as sexual abuse trauma or some medical condition or treatment may be suppressing their hormone levels. These women have a different problem to solve in order to become orgasmic. But for those who are suffering this condition as a result of low or missing testosterone, there's a cure. We promise.

Psychological and Emotional Blocks to Orgasm

It is important to note that independent of physiology, many women need emotional safety that allows them to relax enough to be sexually receptive and let their bodies work through this "natural" experience. This receptivity is emotional and psychological. This is what we mean when we speak of being "in the mood"; our bodies work the way they were designed to. But without emotional and psychological safety, a full sexual experience that includes orgasm may not be possible.

Some women report that their bodies are working well and they are building to the release of an orgasm—and then it just "goes away." This can happen for a number of reasons:

- *Antidepressants,* which are known to inhibit orgasm.

- *Distracted thinking,* including problem solving, worrying, or focusing on some responsibility that needs to be taken care of. This is guaranteed to interrupt "connectivity" and inhibit the orgasmic experience.

- *Emotional resistance* to being sexually responsive can inhibit orgasm.

- *Past traumas* such as sexual abuse or rape can cause some women to "go away" mentally, and hence not be mentally or emotionally present during sexual behaviors. The body will function and work the way it is designed, but the brain protects these women from this experience.

If a woman is not having orgasms, or has never had an orgasm, the first step is to check the levels of testosterone in her system. Second is an evaluation of medicines she may be on. Third, the physician should find out whether or not she has a history of trauma. Fourth, he or she must explore her full medical history and the functioning of her relationship. Many women find that the best answer is a multidisciplinary approach incorporating good medical treatment with good counseling.

The Science of an Orgasm

Some women who are anorgasmic tell us that they do not know for sure if they have ever had an orgasm and ask, "How would I know?" It is useful to discuss this incredible, oxytocin-making, good-feeling process from the scientific perspective of what goes on when someone has an orgasm.

Dr. Beverly Whipple has done extensive research on the brain and physiology of orgasm in women, and she reports that every portion of the brain is engaged in some way in the orgasmic experience. Looking at an MRI as a woman has an orgasm, it is easy to see why they often describe the experience as fireworks going off. Women are aroused to orgasm in three distinct parts of their bodies: the clitoris, the G-spot, and the cervix. Even though the brain is involved in each one, there are localized stimulatory and erotic areas that trigger the release called orgasm. Each of these areas "feels" different when sexual intimacy occurs.

At the surface of the skin, there are sensory nerve bundles that, when stimulated, carry messages to the brain by different "highways." When the clitoris is stimulated, the messages from that area go to the lower levels of the spine and then are transmitted up the central nervous system to the brain. The G-spot and cervix each have their own "highway" to the brain. The sensory bundles that go from these areas approach the central nervous system at differing locations. Most women have areas where most of their orgasms originate, either because of their sexual practices or because of the nerve bundles that are peculiar to their own anatomy. Most often this is the clitoris, which can be stimulated manually, orally, or by pressure during sexual intercourse. Orgasms can be triggered at any or all of the three trigger sites, and it is possible for a woman to have an incredibly powerful orgasm that is triggered at all three locations at the same time!

Physical Causes for Orgasm Loss

Some women who have hysterectomies that include the removal of their cervix will lose one of their three orgasmic sites. If this was the primary or only site from which a woman managed to experience orgasm, she will be devastated. If she is fortunate enough to be able to experience orgasms from the other two sites, she may not even notice the loss.

Orgasms may also fail when there is not enough testosterone. The key here is that testosterone causes the release of nitric oxides. Nitric oxides cause the vascular congestion that leads to swelling of the sexual organs in order to increase the amount of area available for friction. This swollen friction is what physically leads to the release we call orgasm. This testosterone-related process is the same for women and men.

There is also, according to Dr. Whipple's research, a specific peripheral nerve that runs from each of the orgasm sites directly to the brain to signal the release of oxytocin, the overwhelming pleasure chemical that is released in the culmination of the orgasmic experience. If there is damage to these nerves, there is a loss of the powerful sense of completion that we call orgasm.

One of the ways that people "know" that they have orgasms is that they ejaculate. Both men and women can and do ejaculate. Men, especially when they are younger, tend to focus on this single event as the goal of any sexual encounter. As men age, or rather as they mature, their ability to participate in sexual intimacy becomes more about the intimacy and less about the orgasm. Ejaculation is often, but not always, part of an orgasm. It is visible and tangible, but ejaculation is not absolutely necessary for the experience of an orgasm.

In addition to physical and psychological blocks, there can be social inhibitors that we have not discussed because the social complexities that limit sexual behaviors among men and women represent an entirely different field of study. If you are interested in knowing more about this subject, you can search among both sociological and anthropological literature for references.

NONPHYSICAL BARRIERS TO INTIMACY

Thus far, we have been talking about arousal and attraction in mating patterns. Now let's look a little closer at some of the problems that can disrupt or inhibit the sexual expression of intimacy in an established relationship.

Sometimes sexual problems develop due to outside pressures such as money, stress, or life problems. Relationships also unwind when partners discover that after the bloom is off the rose, they do not feel attracted to or very much like each other. Finally, physiological changes in either partner can lead to problems of intimacy and sexual functioning.

So which comes first: depression, or anxiety and the loss of libido? Or is the loss of testosterone the reason libido diminishes? Any or all of these can cause loss or disruption of sexual desire and responsiveness. In many cases the loss of testosterone is the initial cause of the problem. So we have learned to always look behind the symptoms of depression/anxiety to see if there is first and foremost a testosterone problem.

Areas of concern about sexual performance often arise when one of the partners is either overly anxious or overly depressed. One often masks the presence of the other. When you treat depression and there is improvement, often you discover anxiety at a level that disrupts functioning. It can happen the other way as well; you can control the anxiety and discover that the individual is also depressed.

MAYBE I'M JUST NUTS!

Some women with symptoms such as those we have described grow concerned that they are having psychological problems. When they consult a doctor specializing in hormone replacement therapy, they explain that they no longer feel like themselves. They say they have changed on the inside and are not the women they were before all this happened. They feel trapped in bodies that are not theirs, and they cannot find a way to do anything about it.

These women are trying to learn how to operate an unfamiliar system, and they talk about how their desire for everything that once was important to them has gone. They do not desire sex, and they do not enjoy the things they once did, such as going out to a nice restaurant or entertaining friends. They say they feel "gutted" and that their inner self has just gone away. They naturally feel powerless to do anything about it.

They are acutely aware of the change in themselves, and they worry that they are going crazy. Many people in their lives may reinforce that idea, telling them they should be medicated or even institutionalized. Most women are reluctant to mention this to their doctors because of fear that their doctors will agree. They feel broken in a serious way, and on top of that, they feel isolated because no one seems to know why it's happening or what to do about it. Thus, it takes a lot of courage for them to tell a third party what they are going through.

Before they find help, these women who fear loss of their sanity usually attempt to hide their symptoms and their fears. They try for a while to walk through their lives under the radar, in hiding, hoping their husbands and others won't notice. When they gain the courage to actually tell their doctors what is going on, they are very relieved to hear that many other women have described exactly the same problems. They are heartened that there is hope for significant improvement. Yet they are also afraid to believe their problems are treatable and curable with the replacement of just a single hormone that they often did not know they even had.

When Hormones Are Replaced, Why Isn't It All Better?

This is a question many couples ask Brett as a therapist. For some lucky couples, life is better once the hormones are replaced and the libido is rejuvenated. For many others, it is not that simple. Depending on how long their intimacy has atrophied, couples have made adjustments that separate and isolate them from each other on a connected level. They have each made accommodations that allow the marriage to exist and the family to "work," but they have grown apart. This emotional separation is often surrounded by layers of hurt and anger, or even just numbness.

How do you get over this hurt and anger and the adaptive responses you have made to fulfill your life when your partner has not seen or noticed you for a very long time? How do you let go of the old wounds and not use them as ammunition to wound your partner or defend yourself?

Couples have to look at their relationship skills and expectations and work on their abilities to communicate. They must learn how to communicate *first* with themselves in an honest way. Who am I? What do I want? And then they have to take the risk to offer that information to their partner and say, "This is who and what I am and what I want—do you still want me and will you still love me?"

Each partner needs to get to the place where he or she can have this conversation within him- or herself, and then with his or her partner. This often requires the intervention of a therapist who is an expert in communication skills, possesses an understanding of how relationship patterns work, and knows how cultural influences constrict or hamper our abilities to be honest with ourselves and with one another.

As a therapist, Brett finds that many people are not able to talk to their partners about what they like, want, or even fantasize. He often suggests to these couples that they begin by writing fantasy journals, to be kept private from each other and then brought to the sessions. Then he has each of them read just two paragraphs from their journal out loud and talk about what they have said. He asks them to share how it feels to take this risk and reveal some of what they want and what their feelings are about what they have heard. Would they would be willing to "test" or experiment with what they heard?

Finally, he asks if they have any strong adverse reactions to what they have heard. If so, he asks them to stay with those feelings for a little while so together they can explore where they came from and what they mean. These issues can stem from a variety of sources. One of the partners may have a shame-based orientation to sex, a duty-based orientation, or religious limitations that are different from or disappointing to the other partner. People come to sexual encounters with various expectations, understandings of "satisfaction," time cycles, and levels of availability for intimacy, as well as different focal points regarding orgasm and frequency. It can be complex, painful, and frightening when partners are out of sync or on different pages.

A person who has been out of hormonal balance for a period of time may now find herself in a relationship that can be colored by dissatisfaction or lack of desire. During the period she has been distant, the couple may have developed psychological ruts that are difficult to overcome. When they receive hormonal treatment and balance is restored, the status of the relationship will likely change.

Long-standing habits and expectations may have changed for one partner but not the other. It is then Brett's job to clarify each partner's expectations and help them see patterns that prevent them from moving forward and reengaging in the relationship.

Here is a simplistic example of not looking to see whether habits may have changed. When Brett was very young and newly married, he did not like pizza and would not eat it. Many years later, he and his wife were having a conversation about what to order for dinner. She mentioned that she would like to order pizza but that it was not a good choice since he did not like it. He laughed because he had been eating pizza for years, but she had not noticed! She had already labeled him as a non–pizza eater. She had not examined that label carefully for some time or noticed that some of his likes and dislikes had changed.

Eating pizza is an insignificant matter but is illustrative of an important point. Once we have been in a relationship for an extended period of time, our habituation allows us to make pretty accurate assumptions about what our partner thinks, wants, or will say and do. We have become so rhythmically attuned to them that we can make social plans, make decisions about dinner, and know whom to invite and whom to ignore for social plans. We know each other so well that we can complete thoughts, sentences, and jokes for one another. That can be a good and happiness-making confluence in a fulfilling relationship.

There can be problems here, though. Once we have imprinted our perceptions of our partner in our memory, we often stop noticing the changes in their preferences. We assume that they are the same person we married and don't look for changes in their behavior. What if this lack of awareness about changes in our partner's preferences is not restricted to pizza but involves preferences in what they want or like emotionally or sexually? How can we possibly please our loved one if we do not look for or discuss changes in their desires?

A satisfying sex life requires conversation between both partners about the changes in their desires and their goals in sex and pleasure. There is nothing more satisfying than to please your loved one exactly as they desire. On the other hand, our partners cannot read our minds about what we want, so actually saying what we want is often necessary!

For an example of how talking cuts to the chase in relation to squabbles over bedroom preferences, let's consider Pam and Mike's relationship. Pam waited for years to tell Mike that her preference was to wake up on Saturday mornings and have sex when she was relaxed, before the day started. Her husband was astounded that she had never told him that before! Mike had been chasing her around the kitchen trying to get her interested Sunday through Friday, and he was just wasting his time! Now he finally realized that it wasn't *him* she was rejecting, and why she never . . . not once, ever . . . picked up his cue and responded, except on Saturday mornings. If Pam had just discussed her preferences, they could have avoided all of the negative emotions and negotiated a compromise plan.

This is the kind of emotional conundrum that can intensify when habits form over years in order to compensate for hurt, fear, or anxiety. The longer a couple is out of sync sexually, the longer it takes to heal. When we regain the sex drive of our youth, often our partner's old accommodations will need to be challenged and changed. To challenge or change them requires that *both* individuals become aware of them. That takes courage and a willingness to communicate.

Remember, the longer the sexual dissynchrony has gone on, the longer it takes to heal. There are associated issues that grow like weeds around the primary problem of lack of libido: feelings of rejection, anger, and animosity develop and must be addressed. This often requires the help of a licensed counselor trained in resolving these issues. Recovery takes the willingness, time, and effort of both partners to reinvest in the part of the relationship that had been lost.

Brett's patients find it helpful to set aside dedicated, uninterrupted time with their spouses, opportunities to be alone and both discuss their feelings and act on them if they choose. Setting up appointments such as these is a homework assignment many therapists use. William Masters and Virginia Johnson, the pioneering sex experts who established the Masters and Johnson Institute, conducted a compelling study in which they instructed couples to relearn about their partners' physical desires. Their homework was to go home and explore their partners' erotic zones but not have sex. At first the couples were limited to touching nonsexual areas of each other's bodies. More erotic areas were added the following week. Finally, intercourse was allowed. This process forced the couple to find ways to please each other. Inevitably, couples would come back to discuss their "homework" and admit that they could not help having sex . . . and it was great! Success!

A successful process for regaining a fulfilling sex life is different for every couple. The basic idea of communicating desires and needs to one's loved one is difficult, but it is a basic premise for all sexual therapy.

BEHAVIOR PATTERNS

We develop stereotypes for many reasons, not the least of which is that they save us time. We habituate for the same reason. Remember when you were a child and you were trying to learn to tie your shoes? You had to concentrate so hard, and it was a very difficult lesson to learn. You got very frustrated as you tried to master it. But now you can tie your shoes, eat breakfast, watch television, and have a phone conversation all at the same time. The reason you can do this is that you have habituated these behaviors. They are now automatic and reflexive.

We do the same thing in relationships. Have you ever had a phone conversation with your mother and realized that you were not paying any attention at all? You know the rhythms of her speech and of her life. You can talk to her on the phone while you fix dinner, and you can interject an "Oh, my" or a laugh or a "What did he say then?" without much thought. If you actually need to attend to her in some thoughtful and present way, she will signal you by behaving differently from the way she normally does. That change is what gets you to focus. Otherwise you can finish the conversation and hang up without remembering anything she said.

When we move a relationship into commitment or marriage, we automate a pattern of behaving in the relationship. We learn over time to habituate to the pattern we have created and let our awareness of our partner fade into the background. It becomes easy to label the person in our minds: "He doesn't like pizza or white wine. He wants this, that, or the other in the bedroom." We slap on these labels, and we need to remind ourselves that our partner's likes and dislikes evolve and change—just as ours do.

The point here is that we do this with our partners much more than we realize. For example, Brett may start to ask a question and his wife will answer it before he finishes the sentence. She can do this because their lives are quite habituated. Depending on the time, the location, and the topic, she knows the two or three possible things he might say. She even knows all his jokes and can laugh at the punch lines without paying any attention at all. These are good things that help relationships function . . . until all of a sudden they are *not* good things and they do *not* function. When people habituate responses to sexual cueing and requests for intimacy, they are really not attending but simply acting out of habit or responding reflexively. People even reach the point of having sex without paying particular attention to each other. The result: wham, bam, thank you ma'am, and good night! There is no real communication or intimacy.

TDS Raises the Stakes

Habituation at some level is common to every marriage, but when it leads to labeling and assumptions, it can result in very empty, unhappy relationships. If this pattern is compounded by issues of aging, things become more difficult to endure and resolve.

The loss of testosterone and estrogen in particular can compound your feelings of emptiness and unhappiness. When you receive the regenerating effects of bio-identical hormone replacement pellets from your doctor, your physiology will be restored. You will have energy, alertness, and desire. You will be better able to lose weight, increase your stamina, and become sexually interested, which may increase intimacy, or at least the desire for and the expectation of intimacy. The capacity you felt early in your relationship is, or can be, restored.

For some, this is enough. Their bodies work, they rediscover themselves, and life becomes exponentially better and more satisfying. Their sex lives are stimulating and satisfying once again. But for other clients, those who had preexisting patterns of unhappiness and mis- or disconnectedness, these issues will remain. Those couples who had distance in their marriages will still function the same way in their relationships. In these cases, their choices tend to be one of these three options:

1. Get therapy to try to learn new ways to connect and new ways to function with each other . . . in essence, learn to have a new relationship with an old partner.

2. Have their potential and capacity restored, but still not be interested in or responsive to each other.

3. Look for new partners with whom to create "new" relationships.

The clients who choose option one or three have behaviors that tend to fall in patterns. The following case studies illustrate how some clients have worked through these issues and changed their behavior patterns. These client situations represent descriptive patterns and clusters of symptoms; hence the descriptions represent groups of similar clients, not any single individual or couple.

As you read through these examples, you may recognize some aspect of yourself or your partner. This is to be expected. The lines between categories are often fluid. As you read, try to see which pattern fits you *most* of the time. You may see yourself in elements of the other patterns, but you should be able to recognize the predominant one.

Also, it is worth noting that when people look for these patterns, it is often easier for them to identify their partner's strategy or pattern than their own. This is known as denial. If you want to change, you must learn to give up your denial. Then a different future will open for you.

ALAN AND BRENDA

Alan and Brenda are a couple in their 60s. Brenda thought that Alan no longer found her sexually attractive. Alan swore that he loved Brenda and did find her sexually stimulating, but sex itself was just not that great. As they talked about their relationship, Brenda realized that she was willing to respond but never seemed to initiate. Sex had become a chore. Alan realized that it was getting easier to do other things. They were both sad that sex had gone but were learning to adjust to just getting old.

Despite their acceptance of this situation, Alan and Brenda worried that their marriage lacked connectedness. Something was missing, and they wanted it. They feared they might drift away from each other, as they had seen some other couples do. They still loved each other and were willing to try to something new.

Brenda mentioned that some of her friends had been talking about seeing Dr. Maupin for hormone replacement treatments. Her friends were experiencing a vitality that they hadn't felt in a long time. They were beginning to feel a desire for sex again, and their bodies were responsive in ways they had not been since a much younger age. Their husbands were experiencing similar improvements.

Finding similar results, Brenda and Alan noticed increased libido and arousal, but sexual intimacy did not flourish. In therapy, they focused on sex as a process, not as an event. They worked on flirting behaviors and putting effort into new ways of initiating sex, as well as new roles for each of them to improve intimacy and intensity.

Today, Brenda and Alan have begun to find the excitement, energy, and hopefulness of their younger selves. They are in a joyful new phase. It isn't as dismal as "just getting old."

Flirting and Foreplay

Your mind is your most sexual organ. The more you learn to engage it, the greater your sexual intensity and joy will be. Learning to take the time to arouse each other verbally and mentally adds much power to the connection. Couples who begin early in the day to call each other and say sexy things, leave notes for each other in their briefcases, and whisper about what they want to do build a level of sexual tension that can help make their encounter, when it happens, much more powerful. Work on spending time touching, kissing, and stroking throughout the evening while delaying actual intercourse. Think about having sex in different or unusual (for you) places so that it does not become routine and automatic.

MARGARET

Margaret divorced her husband when she was 55 years old and initially did not need or want the company of someone of the opposite sex. Margaret and her ex-husband had fewer and fewer sexual encounters after she was in her mid-40s, and she sure didn't miss it! She believed that was normal, but her husband disagreed. Sex became just one of the many things they disagreed about.

Margaret was lonely after a year of the single life, and she was not as welcome in her social circle of married couples anymore. She found life to be empty and somewhat boring. She hoped that dating would help her be accepted again by her married friends and add more enjoyment to her life but was concerned about the issue of sex. As it turned out, dating reignited that old problem; she still was not interested in sex, even though she did want to find a companion. This issue caused her a lot of anxiety and delayed her accepting dates. She knew sex would eventually become a problem.

Margaret met a man at a church event and went to dinner with him, and a few dates later she ended up in bed with him. This was the miserable experience she had feared. She was dry and had pain during intercourse, as well as after. She felt like she had been rubbed raw with sandpaper. The pain was one thing, but she felt nothing else was pleasant about the encounter either, and she could not wait to flee this very nice guy's house. She delayed dating again and finally confided her situation to one of her friends who also had reentered the dating life. Her friend advised her to get her hormones checked because, in her friend's words, "What is happening is not normal, and there is treatment for it! I had my estrogen and testosterone replaced, and I feel like I felt before my first marriage!"

After seeing her friend's hormone doctor, she began to feel like her old self again. In fact, she couldn't remember the last time she had felt aroused or "sexy"; it had been so long. Her confidence in the dating process began to increase with her libido, and her fear abated. She decided that before going through the embarrassment of another failed sexual encounter, she would explore and experiment. She asked her younger friends about vibrators because she wanted to "practice" before her next encounter. By masturbating she discovered what she liked and wanted from sex. By getting some help from hormones and adapting to a new world of dating, Margaret had all the tools she needed to have a fulfilling second half of her life!

TOM AND NANCY

Tom and Nancy are not married. They met three years ago when Nancy began dating, after her divorce from Claude. Six months later, they moved in together. In the beginning, their intimate lives were all either of them wanted, but TDS hit Nancy hard a year ago. She felt Tom begin to pull away and did not know what to do. Sex had become something she was doing because she wanted to make him happy, not because she desired it. She went through the motions and did the things she thought he wanted; she even faked orgasms. (Nancy said that she would just get tired and lose interest but did not want to hurt his feelings.)

Tom was different from Claude because he "knew" something had changed. He was looking for intimacy and not just sex. When Nancy started showing signs of not being an engaged participant, he questioned her to discover what was going on. Tom wanted her to stay connected and do something about getting "real" again.

Tom was a passionate and considerate lover. He actually wanted Nancy to feel that he loved her and was paying attention to her for her pleasure. When Nancy went through TDS, she could not feel those things anymore. Tom became demanding but not just about sex—about intimacy! "This has to be fixed or we won't make it," he said. Nancy was very surprised that he knew the things he knew about how she was feeling. Claude had never been aware of her in that way.

She did not know where to turn or what to do. She asked some of her girl-friends what they thought. Her friends recommended that she go to a hormone doctor to see if that would help. They had heard about testosterone replacement helping people get their mojo back—maybe it could help Nancy.

The Challenge of Therapy Is Combining Hormonal Replacement with Relationship Healing

Relationships take work; they don't just happen. Intimacy is much more than just lust or magical thinking. It may start with infatuation, but infatuation does not last. When it eventually diminishes, it must resolve itself into something deeper and more meaningful: something we call intimacy.

When a woman's body ages, she feels the negative impact physically in the language of love, which is naturally one of the most important intimate communication skills. When the body begins to slow down sexually, if partners are not open and communicating, if partners have not learned how to talk to each other and learned how to communicate love and affection outside of sexual contact, they lose a connectedness. Then the partners get angry and hurt, and they isolate themselves from intimacy and friendship.

This does not have to happen!

The body does not have to change this way. With the hormone replacement treatments that are now available, people can guard against this decline. They can then focus on maintaining their most intimate friendship with all the blessings of full physical contact.

Hopefully, the discussion of libido and relationships in this chapter has given you enough information to understand how important sex is to our lives and the quality of our relationships. When libido is lost and relationships suffer, seek treatment. It is our hope that the following chapter will allay any fears you may have about replacing your testosterone. We hope you are bold enough to replace your testosterone and get your 30-something sex drive back. It is worth it! As you will discover in the next chapter, the libido is only one of the many benefits of replacing testosterone.

After focusing on sex and libido, it is time to examine testosterone and its impact on or involvement in the symptoms that so many women experience as they enter their 40s and beyond. In the next chapter, we will take a symptom-by-symptom look at blood tests, fatigue, insomnia, anxiety, and depression and a host of other presenting issues that women go to their doctors about. We will touch on some of the standard responses women receive, and we will emphasize the role testosterone plays in each of these presenting problems. As you read, you will find yourself identifying with problems you have experienced or that women you know have shared with you, and you will be relieved to know that there is help that is affordable, safe, and practical.

Now that you have looked at the results of your questionnaire and focused on what might be causing you difficulty, it is time to understand how the loss of testosterone impacts us as we age. Without testosterone we become susceptible to a host of illnesses and ailments commonly identified with aging. Many of these illnesses affect the quality of our lives. They are costly because they limit our mobility, our ability to live independently, and our ability to function in our daily lives. These illnesses require medicines that are expensive, have problematic side effects, and are accompanied by limitations and discomforts. You can avoid most of these problems if you decide to replace your testosterone. Let's see how this may apply to you.

CHAPTER 5

THE SYMPTOMS OF TESTOSTERONE DEFICIENCY SYNDROME

Now that you've answered the first set of questionnaires and suspect that you have symptoms of testosterone deficiency, you're ready to learn about each of your hormone-loss symptoms in detail. This will provide you with more information about the stages of hormonal deficiency and help you determine their causes without blood tests. Although final diagnosis of TDS should be confirmed with blood tests, understanding the part testosterone plays in your symptomology will help you discuss your history with your hormone doctor.

We will examine each of these symptoms individually, and we'll also explore the relationship between testosterone loss and the symptoms, including how hormone replacement alone can help you avoid the associated illnesses—and even save you money on the medicines you may now be using to treat them. We will be looking at issues like low libido, fatigue, insomnia, anxiety and depression, and migraines and other headache types. We will also examine body composition changes that occur when testosterone levels drop. We'll address issues such as cellulite, memory loss and cognition, Alzheimer's, dry eyes, and exercise intolerance, all of which are impacted negatively as testosterone is lost.

LOSS OF SEX DRIVE

In Chapter 4, we discussed societal and relationship reactions to testosterone and libido loss. Here we delve deeper into the medical information regarding loss of sex drive because so many people identify this symptom as an indication of TDS. The path to grasping the truth about testosterone's importance to you and solving your testosterone deficiency can be found in the research of several medical specialties.

Many studies of the last ten years have been directed at the problem of lost libido in middle-aged women but most have not isolated the hormone testosterone as either cause or treatment. The encouraging news is that the numbers of such studies have increased over the last few years, but unfortunately, the results are not being published in the journals that are read by gynecologists, the specialists in women's hormones.

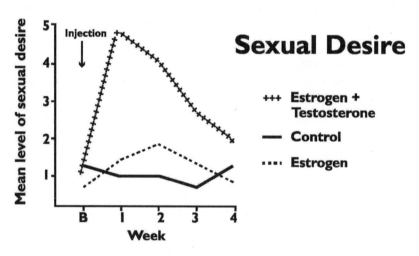

Injection of estrogen + testosterone, the placebo (control), or estrogen alone, occurs at the baseline ("B") stage. The injection lasts for about four weeks, at which time another injection is given.

Dr. Sherwin compared three hormone groups to investigate which hormone replacement caused the greatest improvement in libido, sexual fantasies, and sexual arousal. The chart shown is her results with sexual arousal scores after an injection of estrogen + testosterone, the placebo (control), or estrogen alone. The hormone injections last for about four weeks, at which time another injection is given. The results reveal that women's sexual desire (measured by grading the woman's own determined level of libido) was most affected by the combination of estradiol and testosterone in intramuscular injection form, and that estrogen given as an intramuscular (im) injection did not have a significant effect on sexual desire. It was equal to or slightly better than doing nothing. This is evidence that supports the belief that the controlling hormone for women's libido is testosterone—and not estrogen alone, as OB/GYNs have been trained to believe.

Dr. Sherwin used this graph to emphasize the importance of testosterone to women's sexuality. As testosterone is metabolized and levels drop so too does libido. It is not clear why libido goes up in the control group in the third week. Sherwin's study does not conclude anything about that.

Here's the important point. Sex is not magic, though it can often feel like it is. Sex is *science!* This is hard to believe because it seems to undermine the idea of romance. Romance, however, is simply a derivative of the chemical changes the body experiences when sexual energy is abundant. If that energy fails, romance, desire, and sex all collapse. But because sex is science and not magic, we can fix the problem!

Accurately Diagnosing TDS-Related Libido Loss

Richard let it all out. "Doc, you are the last chance for our marriage. I am not living without sex for the rest of my life. She won't even touch me, and beyond that she acts like she doesn't need me anymore! If this doesn't work, I'm gone!"

"I love my wife," he continued, fighting back tears, "but I feel horrible about myself because she doesn't want me anymore. I've given her flowers

and taken her on vacation in an effort to rekindle our love. She tries, but I can tell she doesn't like sex anymore. What am I doing wrong?"

This scenario is played out in the office all the time. Couples who are bold enough often come in together, if only to satisfy the one still interested in sex. They usually believe, and not incorrectly, that seeking help will restore marital harmony and sexual satisfaction. In short, sex—or more specifically, the loss of sex—is one of the biggest motivators for women and their husbands to seek testosterone replacement treatment.

For a regular doctor hearing this complaint, it would be hard to tell whether Richard's wife has lost her sexuality because of a physical, social, or psychological problem. It is common medical knowledge that numerous habits and medications—including drinking alcohol, smoking, and taking many antidepressants, corticosteroids, and high blood pressure medications—can decrease the level or activity of testosterone, thereby decreasing libido, intensity of desire, and performance. Alcohol consumption can affect a normally healthy sexual desire by relaxing inhibitions and increasing the likelihood of engaging in sexual activity, but the flip side is that alcohol dulls the senses and the neurotransmitters, so often sexual performance is blunted or dysfunctional.

As a physician focused on hormones, Kathy has an easier time than most doctors in determining whether a patient's loss of sexual drive is the result of testosterone loss as opposed to a psychological problem or conflict in the marriage. She asks her patients the following questions that help her confirm testosterone deprivation as the culprit.

- Are you over 38 or have you had your ovaries removed?
- Is your best creative energy spent thinking up excuses to avoid having sex with your husband or partner?
- Do you wonder why you ever considered sex interesting?

- Does the thought of your lover touching you make you cringe?
- Do you distract yourself by itemizing your shopping list while you are having sex?
- Is it true that you are not sexually attracted to *anyone?*

If you answered "yes" to most of these, you are most likely experiencing loss of sexual desire (libido) from testosterone deprivation—which of course means you can get it back!

Factors Affecting Libido	
INCREASE LIBIDO	**DECREASE LIBIDO**
Arginine (an amino acid)	Aging >40
Attention deficit disorder medications	Alcohol addiction
Breast stimulation	Androgen insensitivity
Dopamine (Parkinson's meds)	Antidepressants
Estradiol (nonoral)	Birth control pills
Genetics	Blood pressure medicines
Growth hormone	Breastfeeding
HCG (human chorionic gonadotropin)	Cholesterol statins
Oxytocin (neurosteroid)	Diabetes
Testosterone	Mania medications
Thyroid medications	Obesity
	Oral estrogens
	Prolactin
	Removal of ovaries
	Smoking
	Stress and steroid medications
	Stroke

Testosterone Levels Vary by Individual

Adult men have ten times as much testosterone as women, but women have three times as much testosterone as estrogen, the hormone that is normally associated with women. These differing levels of testosterone actually determine our very gender, which, of course, determines our identity, our place in the world, and how we are raised and treated by our family and society. These differing testosterone levels are also responsible for the basic neurological differences between men and women. Testosterone is fundamental and important to who we are.

Within these gender-specific norms, genetics determine testosterone levels from individual to individual. These varying levels explain why sex drives vary and why some people may be publically sexual in every part of their life while others may not consider sexuality to be essential to who they are.

"I'm worried that if I have my testosterone replaced I will be too sexual for my husband. Neither of us has a voracious sexual drive, and I'm happy the way things are," said Amy, age 54. Amy had come in to the office because she had other symptoms of testosterone loss and was resistant to taking testosterone. She was worried that she would develop a higher sex drive than her husband, Fred.

Amy and Fred had genetically determined lower-than-normal sex drives, so their blood levels and receptor sites were below average. This was "normal" for them, and they desired to maintain equally low libidos. In terms of replacement, this becomes a dosage issue, one that your body takes care of for you naturally before you get TDS. This is an important issue that your hormone doctor must consider when replacing testosterone.

Masters and Johnson undertook the most extensive sex research in modern times and taught that *sexual appetite* was much like the appetite for food, varying from individual to individual. The appetite analogy can be helpful in thinking about how we approach sex. Think about how you would eat, how often, and how much if you had your choice. When we enter a relationship we tend to adapt to our partner as to how, what, and when we eat. That is exactly what we should do with sexual appetite. Based on our partner's appetite and our own, we should find middle ground for our sexual activity. It's important to talk with your partner about how often each of you wants to have sex, for how long, and what it consists of. Then you should reach a compromise that is acceptable to both individuals. A sexual activity level somewhere between the two sets of appetites is the ideal plan for sexual activity.

If you have low testosterone and low libido you can replace testosterone and improve your libido. However, if you have other symptoms of testosterone deficiency and do not want to have a heightened sex drive for some reason, you can manage this with lower dosage levels of testosterone.

FATIGUE

Did you know that fatigue is one of the most common symptoms that brings women to the doctor's office? It is also one of most elusive symptoms to diagnose. It can result from a busy life, a virus, a hormonal imbalance from a recent pregnancy or surgery, or a blood disorder as common as anemia or as dangerous as leukemia. Needless to say, one of the causes of severe fatigue is a loss of testosterone.

Because there are many potential causes of fatigue, it is important to have a full medical evaluation to rule out the most dangerous and most common causes of that symptom. The most common physical causes of fatigue include:

- Anemia
- Cardiac arrhythmia and heart failure
- Chronic fatigue caused by the mononucleosis virus
- Depression*
- Hypoglycemia (low blood sugar)*
- Hypopituitary (low pituitary) hormones
- Hypothyroidism (low thyroid hormone)*
- Insomnia; sleep disorders leading to daytime fatigue

- Lack of exercise*
- Lack of testosterone
- Medications (beta blockers, hypertension medications, sedatives, and antidepressants)
- Poor diet; lack of protein, vitamins, and overall nutrition
- Stress and the hormonal imbalance that comes from it (high cortisol)
- Untreated attention deficit disorder and attention deficit hyperactivity disorder (ADD and ADHD)

* These may be triggered by low testosterone.

In their younger years, women often felt fatigued because they were overbooked or ate poorly, spending time caring for their families instead of themselves. The "tired" they experience these days *feels* different. This low-testosterone fatigue is a feeling of being *bone tired*. They crawl to bed and wake up tired, and nothing makes it better . . . not even sleep!

Jenna had circles under her eyes, and she slumped down in her chair. "I'm so tired. I'm a nurse, so I'm used to working hard and feeling sleep deprived. But it's different now that I'm in my 40s. It's so bad that all I can do is work and go home and go to bed. I never feel like doing anything but sleeping—I'm not even hungry! On the weekends I sleep 12 hours a night and still wake up tired. I take naps when I can and stay up for a few hours before I crash again. My other doctors tell me I'm healthy, but I don't feel healthy! I feel so depressed. Something is not right."

After Jenna's blood work was completed and we had ruled out major illnesses, we discovered that her testosterone was nonexistent! Two months after her testosterone pellets were inserted, she was back to her old self and her energy returned in full force. She looked and felt better and was on her way to getting her life back.

"I was a shell of my former self. Testosterone pellets changed my life," said Jenna. *"I feel like I've awakened from a long sleep. I feel better than I did at 35. Not only do I have my life back, but I am now the person I always wanted to be, and I'm living my best life!"*

In the early stages of testosterone deficiency prior to menopause, adding DHEA, an ingredient secreted from the adrenal glands (in doses of 5 to 25 mg per day), to increase testosterone production by the ovaries helps improve testosterone levels—as long as the ovaries are present. If the ovaries have been removed, DHEA cannot make more testosterone because the ovary is the "factory" that produces it. Also, the ovary does not make testosterone in any measurable amounts after menopause, so DHEA will not help at that stage. So, after ovaries are removed or at the onset of menopause, the only way to improve testosterone and energy levels is through replacement. This in turn stimulates the production of the other hormones that give us energy in the following ways:

- Cortisol improves usable energy, adrenaline, and blood pressure and helps us tolerate stress.
- Growth hormone increases metabolism so we burn calories, generate heat, and lose fat.
- Insulin improves the use of blood sugar to make energy and decreases fatigue.
- Norepinephrine, the neurohormone, stimulates our brain and makes us feel energetic, awake, and motivated.
- Melatonin improves restful sleep and therefore makes us more awake during the day.
- Oxytocin improves sexual energy.
- Serotonin improves mood and mental energy.

Testosterone is the one hormone that can fill up a woman's tank with energy by stimulating the production of other hormones that disappear when testosterone is depleted. When fatigue accompanied by the absence of testosterone is treated by replacing the testosterone, energy usually returns within a month.

Other hormones decrease as women age, and they develop habits that cause fatigue, but testosterone is the one hormone replacement that makes the most difference in their energy after age 40.

INSOMNIA

"No matter what I try, I can't sleep!" Carole lamented. She had turned 40 earlier in the year, and she never used to have this problem. "I wake up at 2:30 every morning and can't go back to sleep. When I do fall back to sleep, it's usually around 4:30 A.M., and I have one hour to get rest before I have to get up and go to work. I have been given sleeping pills, which help me sleep a little more, but I still wake up exhausted. I barely make it through the day. In the afternoons I drink coffee to stay awake, but I still feel tired. I am at my wit's end!"

Fatigue and insomnia are two different issues. We may have fatigue as a result of insomnia, but we can also develop fatigue without insomnia. Insomnia leaves us too tired to enjoy life and leads to lowered immunity, higher risk of accidents, and weakened productivity. Interestingly, women have a higher prevalence of insomnia than men by a 2-to-1 ratio, which follows the gender difference in testosterone deficiency. Women lose testosterone ten years before men and have a tenth of the total testosterone men have throughout their reproductive lives.

Sleepless in the OR

The ability to work without sleep has historically been a requirement the medical profession placed on young physicians, despite their obvious loss of performance after the 12th hour of alertness. Only recently has lack of sleep been officially associated with poor quality work and mistakes made by doctors in training. Thankfully, medical residents currently in training have limits on their work hours, but most practicing physicians were trained in the old system when doctors considered the ability to stay awake a badge of honor. Unfortunately, this makes them less likely to consider a lack of sleep important. It is no wonder, then, that when patients complain of insomnia, their doctors often ignore their complaints. But insomnia is a risk factor for poor health and should be attended to and treated.

If, like Carole, you have developed insomnia for the first time in your middle-aged years, you are not alone. Want some proof? Watch a little television at 2 A.M. and count the number of infomercials and paid TV shows directed toward women. You'll see them talk about cosmetics, clothing, hair styling products, shoe and purse organizers, antiaging creams, and so on. The advertising agencies of the world know that women in the over-40 age group aren't sleeping!

There are many prescription and over-the-counter (OTC) sleep aids available, but these only treat the symptom of sleeplessness and not the root cause. Also, most of us need the mental and physical healing that takes place during deep sleep, but sadly, sleep aids and prescriptions don't induce normal deep sleep.

The proven initial cause of insomnia after age 40 in women and age 50 in men is lower testosterone, as published in literature from the American Academy of Neurology in its journal, *Neurology*. These studies reveal the role of testosterone in regaining the four stages of sleep necessary for us to feel rested and refreshed every morning. The only cure for age-related insomnia is the replacement of testosterone.

TDS-Related Insomnia

If you want to figure out whether your sleeplessness is caused by TDS, compare your insomnia to the following characteristics of insomnia related to TDS:

- Lack of dreaming and deep sleep
- No previous history of insomnia before age 35
- Waking between 2:00 and 3:30 A.M. and being unable to fall back to sleep until 4 to 5 A.M.
- Waking fatigued and not feeling refreshed

Testosterone aids with deep, restful sleep and healing rapid eye movement (REM) sleep. During REM sleep we repair our cells, work out our psychological problems, and rest our brain, refreshing it for the day to come. Sounds amazing, doesn't it?

Without adequate testosterone, we go to sleep easily and progress through the first three stages of sleep. But when it comes time to enter stage 4, REM sleep, we wake up, never or only briefly entering the last and most important stage. This process recurs again and again through the night and leaves the insomniac poorly rested and unable to be fully awake during the day.

Let's compare the loss of stage 4 sleep with the plight of the Greek god, Sisyphus, who was eternally doomed to push a heavy boulder up a mountain. Once he finally reached the top, he was forced to watch the boulder slip away and roll back down the mountain. Then he had to push it up again. Most patients say that going through the preparatory stages of sleep—stages 1 through 3—only to wake up and go back to stage 1, creates the same feeling as if they were Sisyphus. Night after night, it never ends!

This particular type of TDS-related insomnia only responds to replacing the hormones we are missing. Testosterone is the hormone that creates restful sleep by replenishing the neurotransmitters that promote both REM and non-REM deep sleep.

"Testosterone replacement has made such a positive difference in daily life. I no longer suffer from migraine headaches, and I sleep through the night feeling rested," Carole exclaimed during our follow-up consultation a month later. "My energy has dramatically increased! One hormone has now replaced three drugs for sleep and migraine headaches."

Most patients need only testosterone to re-create normal sleep patterns, yet in some cases, replacing testosterone is not enough. Progesterone replacement may be necessary to stimulate the secretion of serotonin, a neurotransmitter in the brain that creates relaxation. You should discuss this with your doctor if you find that testosterone alone hasn't done the trick for you.

Long-Term Insomnia Causes Symptoms of Sleep Deprivation

Long-term lack of sleep can change our personality and make us physically ill. This is illustrated every day in the lives of insomniacs who find that lack of sleep begins to affect their relationships, sex drive, mood, and job performance and impairs their immune system so they get sick more often.

Those women who prefer the hands-off approach to hormone replacement and medicine are prone to ignore their insomnia until it leads to other symptoms or illness. But think about this: having your hormones intact is the most normal thing you can experience, and living without them is simply not healthy. If you accept insomnia and avoid testosterone replacement, you will most likely watch your body and mind deteriorate as you head toward more and more sickness. It takes about ten years after your first symptoms of insomnia-related TDS before you begin to see your health deteriorate, so use the knowledge that researchers have given us and help yourself prevent future illness!

ASK BRETT

"I have have trouble focusing and sitting still, and I am easily distracted. I have trouble sleeping at night, so I'm always tired and foggy headed. My husband and I fight a lot because I am so scattered and tired. I often forget to take care of important tasks.

"I have never been diagnosed with ADD or ADHD. I have had a hysterectomy, but other than that I do not have any medical issues that I am aware of. What should I do?" — Debbie, 43

Debbie, I would first suggest you talk to a physician and get a check-up to make sure that your attention and fatigue issues do not have an underlying medical cause. You should also look at your stress levels and your schedule. Are there any immediate triggers for stress, sleeplessness, or concentration issues that you can identify? It is entirely possible that the issues you are suffering would benefit from hormone replacement therapy, but it is equally possible that these are legitimate stand-alone concerns that require their own intervention and treatment strategy. Begin by eliminating possibilities from the easiest to the hardest.

Sit down and talk to your husband about your concerns. Calmly and patiently explain that what you are experiencing is legitimate and documentable, not to mention treatable. You do not need to suffer because of his, or anyone else's, limited point of view.

The Outcome of Testosterone Replacement for Insomnia

Once women begin testosterone therapy, wonderful things begin to happen with their sleep:

- Daytime fatigue is relieved.
- Depression and anxiety decrease.
- Energy levels improve.
- Immune response improves.
- Mental tasks become easier.
- Restful sleep returns.
- Weight loss begins because of increased melatonin levels from sleep.
- You progressively feel like yourself of old.

Replacement of testosterone improves many things, and sleep is a critical quality-of-life issue women need to pay attention to in order to achieve health and regain youthful energy, mood, and productivity.

ANXIETY AND DEPRESSION

Anxiety and depression represent two of the most common complaints in doctors' offices all over America. Both symptoms are much more common in women than in men, generally because men tend to self-medicate with alcohol and are hence often diagnosed with alcoholism instead.

The terminology alone is confusing because anxiety and depression both have definitions that are socially vague and simultaneously medically precise. When your son is "anxious" about a final exam or your daughter is "depressed" because she did not make the cheerleading squad, they are not necessarily clinically anxious or depressed, and everyone understands that. When they experience extremely intense or long-standing anxiety or depression, however, they may be moving from a social situation to a medical condition.

Common Signs of Depression

- Change in appetite
- Excessive worrying
- Hopelessness
- Irritability
- Lack of energy
- Lack of libido
- Loss of motivation
- Sadness
- Waking at 2 to 3 A.M. every night

In focusing on the medical definitions of depression, we need to differentiate between symptoms and causes. Symptoms are those behavioral or experiential manifestations that people "feel" and respond to. They tell us that something is wrong. Doctors obtain the symptoms when they take a history from the patient. The patient will tell the doctor how she feels and what she is afraid of, and the doctor looks for an illness-related medical cause.

Common symptoms falling under the umbrella label of "depression" include interrupted sleep (usually waking around 2 A.M.), irritability, and poor concentration. Most women who suffer from depression ask, "Is this all there is?" People who are depressed believe that their happiest experiences are not fulfilling or enjoyable. They believe life is dull and humorless. They often feel hopeless. True depression is evident in the dull and emotionless eyes of the depressed patient.

Two Kinds of Medical Depression

The common use of the word *depression* dilutes its true medical meaning. Clinical depression is more than just situational sadness. Everyone goes through periods when they feel depressed: the death of a loved one, a job loss, or a sudden illness can all be contributors. Clinical depression involves at least three consecutive months of a daily low mood. It's due to a chemical imbalance, with the final biologic effect resulting in a deficit in the amount and absorption of serotonin, a chemical produced in the brain that allows us to maintain our cheery mood.

In terms of cause, there are two types of depression: exogenous and endogenous. Exogenous depression occurs when an outside factor leads to these feelings, such the job loss mentioned earlier. Endogenous depression is caused by physical imbalances within the chemistry of the body. Hormonally triggered depression is an example of this kind of depression.

If the situation that causes an exogenous depression is traumatic enough, or if the situation lasts for an extended period of time—a prolonged or life-threatening illness, for example—it can become endogenous, because neurotransmitters such as serotonin become depleted, which causes a chemical imbalance in the brain that we experience as depression. One thing that is clear: life events impact us more severely after we turn 40, after which time it is much more difficult to bounce back.

When women's lives are going well and there is no identifiable reason for these feelings, the cause is usually endogenous. They are simply losing their hormones and with them go the neurotransmitters, such as serotonin, that have supplied the energy and emotional stamina that allowed them to withstand the stresses of life. Again, the age of 40 seems to be critical because, frequently, the initial trigger in women over 40 is the loss of testosterone and thyroid hormone that makes them much more susceptible to chemical depression.

Treatment Options for Testosterone-Related Depression

Because there are multiple causes for depression and many hormones involved, it is obviously an intricate system that keeps us smiling. Physiological, emotional, or psychological events can all contribute to the symptoms we call anxiety or depression, so isolating specific causes can be challenging. As a result, physicians often find themselves treating the symptoms without really knowing the cause. Usually they treat with an antidepressant, but this isn't always the best course of action. Some women can avoid having to take antidepressants, with their attendant costs and side effects, by having their hormones replaced to premenopausal levels.

In either case, an assessment needs to be made about the appropriateness of medicines. If you need to take an antidepressant, you should know that generally it is recommended for at least six months to a year before trying to come off it. There are many reasons for this, and you should carefully discuss antidepressants with your physician. Only a physician who is licensed and trained in the diagnosis of mood disorders, like a psychologist or a professional counselor, can diagnose depression accurately. The treatment can involve medications to replace missing serotonin or the hormones that may be

THE SECRET FEMALE HORMONE

deficient. In general, counseling is also needed to assist in behavioral changes to prevent recurrences of this condition.

ASK BRETT

"I have been diagnosed as bipolar. Sometimes I am depressed, and sometimes I am manic. I do not really know if I have an anxiety disorder, too, because the mania and depression are so overwhelming. My libido is low, and I think that is contributing to my depression. Would testosterone replacement help me?" —Betty, 56

Betty, if you suffer from hormone loss, particularly testosterone loss, then replacing it may help you. In particular, the portions of your distress that manifest in loss of libido and sexual nonresponsiveness would likely be improved.

Testosterone can work very well to help regulate depression but does not work well to limit the mania associated with bipolar disorder. The mania has to be regulated by additional medications.

If you are considering testosterone replacement, it is necessary that you speak with your physician about being bipolar and that you continue to work with a psychiatrist throughout this process. Testosterone replacement will not in and of itself "cure" you from the issues you have with being bipolar. The physical components of the imbalances may be repaired with hormone replacement, but the emotional and behavioral issues will need to be addressed with additional medicine and ongoing therapy.

Anxiety, Depression, or Both?

Another frustrating complication is that anxiety is often masked by severe depression. In this scenario, after the depression is treated and diminishes, the anxiety becomes visible. This can also happen the other way around: we can discover depression after treating anxiety. If you are experiencing anxiety attacks, if you are constantly waiting for the other shoe to fall, or if you startle easily and have trouble focusing, you may be suffering from generalized anxiety disorder (GAD). There are medicines designed specifically to treat anxiety, and there are also behaviorally focused treatments to manage and reduce it. If anxiety symptoms are caused or exacerbated by low levels of testosterone, replacement of your hormones may mean you will not need antianxiety meds. Be aware that there's a distinction between generalized anxiety and other forms of anxiety, such as panic attacks or phobias.

Hormonal Imbalances and Serotonin Production

As we mentioned, serotonin is that magical chemical that helps us sustain our good mood and positive outlook. Testosterone stimulates the production of serotonin and the secretion in the brain of norepinephrine, which gives us energy, improves mood, and heightens concentration. When we're stressed, however, cortisol levels increase, and this results in testosterone levels dropping quickly to a much lower level. This explains why we feel worse during times of stress.

Depression may also be triggered by deficient levels of hormones other than testosterone, such as progesterone, thyroid hormones, and melatonin. If you ask most PMS patients about depression, they say that they are depressed for two out of every four weeks each month. Generally, this type of depression results from low levels of testosterone and progesterone that occur during the second half of the menstrual cycle. These hormones stabilize the brain and improve serotonin levels. Testosterone is secreted throughout the menstrual cycle, but progesterone is made only in the second half of the cycle. When the ovary makes a lower than necessary amount of progesterone, estradiol increases; this imbalance causes the serotonin to drop, resulting in depression. This problem is much more likely to happen in women who are testosterone deprived, so PMS and depression are generally more severe after age 40.

Your thyroid hormones are also responsible for your mood. When there is a deficiency in thyroid hormones for any reason, patients can feel depressed. This type of depression is generally described as a type of slow motion or fatigue and depression combined; it feels like you're walking through a bowl full of Jell-O.

The takeaway from all of this is that anxiety and depression are treatable. You do not have to suffer without hope. There is a range of possible helping steps. Antidepressants, hormone replacement, therapy, and yoga are just some of the things that can bring relief.

MIGRAINE HEADACHES AND TESTOSTERONE

Have you ever had a migraine? If you're not sure, then there's a good chance you haven't! Migraine headaches are so painful they make it practically impossible to get anything done. All you want to do is lie down in the dark until one passes.

Migraine headaches are rarely associated with hormones, yet they are intimately involved with women's hormonal milieu. This causes a problem for doctors because neurologists care for headaches, gynecologists take care of women's hormones, and research on migraines and hormonal effects are found in the subspecialty of endocrinology. It is easy to understand the confusion, but a few specialty-crossing researchers have made the connection between testosterone and migraines.

We have been able to extinguish this type of migraine headache so effectively in patients that people come from as far as Australia, Japan, and Germany to get testosterone pellets just to eliminate their migraines. Locally, several neurologists specializing in headache treatment send their female patients over age 35 to Kathy if they have been unable to remedy their headaches with traditional medical treatments.

Ruling out Nonmigraine Headaches

If you think you may be suffering from migraines, the first thing to do is to make sure your headaches are, in fact, true migraines. Other headaches can be mistaken for them, and we doctors must rule out the headaches that are dangerous, such as one resulting from a brain tumor or from very high blood pressure.

To rule out these other possibilities, you need a neurological checkup with a physical exam that includes measuring blood pressure and pulse. You may also want to have an electroencephalogram (EEG), which tests your brain waves. Your doctor may also recommend an MRI and/or CT scan of your brain, and possibly a carotid Doppler test, which uses sound waves to measure the flow of blood through the large carotid arteries that supply blood to the brain. These tests will give your doctor enough information to determine whether or not your headache is life threatening, the cause or trigger that begins the headache, and finally, the best treatment plan.

Other Kinds of Headaches

- Allergy
- Brain tumor
- High blood pressure
- Muscle tension
- Sinus congestion
- TMJ (temporomandibular joint) pain

There are many less medically serious causes of headaches, but they are just as painful and disruptive. All recurrent headaches should be evaluated and treated by a neurologist or other qualified physician. Headaches may result from muscle tension, sinus problems, grinding or clenching your teeth (which causes pain in the upper jaw—TMJ), high blood pressure, abnormal blood vessels in the brain, or migraines from swelling of the blood vessels in the brain.

Most of us have experienced a muscle tension headache at some point in our lives. Women tend to hold stress in their necks and backs so often have a lifetime of muscle tension headaches. These headaches begin at the base of the skull in the back of the neck and may reach the forehead region. They can be treated with muscle relaxants and mild pain relievers. For a more natural treatment, alternating ice and heat is a good at-home treatment. Massages or physical therapy can relieve and prevent these pesky headaches without medication. Most specialists in "active release" massage and physical therapy will offer at-home exercises that can prevent recurrences.

Sinus headaches are common in patients who have a deviated septum in their nose or have genetically small sinuses that don't have room to accommodate congestion or changes in barometric pressure. Allergies are often the trigger for this type of headache. Sinuses are just large holes in your facial bones like "caves" with a single exit, located in the front of your face. When blocked, they cause pain around the eyes and cheeks. To identify whether this is your problem, tap your forehead or cheeks when you have a headache; if there is pain, this is generally a sinus headache. A trip to your ENT (ear, nose, and throat doctor) can help you determine whether you need surgery to open your sinuses or correct your nasal septum. These specialists generally order an X-ray of some type. Treatments for sinus headaches include antihistamines, Claritin, antibiotics, hot packs, nasal steroids, and the very clever, inexpensive neti pot that lets you to rinse out your sinuses to clear them of debris.

Allergy headaches accompany other allergy symptoms and center in the same area as the sinus headache. Kathy always sends patients who have nasal drainage, coughing, sneezing, rashes, or food allergies with sinuslike headaches to an allergist for skin tests before treating them with testosterone replacement. Often allergy headaches can be relieved by getting allergy shots or avoiding certain foods. Nasal cortisone medications relieve sinus allergy headaches as well.

TMJ headaches create pain around the "hinge" of the jaw near the temples. This headache is from a muscle spasm and inflammation of the joint from grinding teeth, either during sleep or all the time. Dentists care for this type of headache by fitting patients with a mouth guard to wear at night.

Migraines: Where They Come from and How to Combat Them

You can thank your family for your migraines. They're genetic! Basically, they are caused by swollen veins in the skull that expand because of an increased excitability of the nerves in the brain. Because the skull doesn't stretch, the swollen veins increase the pressure in the skull and this causes pain.

Migraine headaches are often accompanied by a visual "aura" of lights and flashes prior to the pain, one-sided (brain hemisphere) pain, sensitivity to light, feelings of nausea and/or vomiting, and failure to respond to Tylenol or aspirin.

Most women with migraines describe their headache with their hands, placing them over one eye and one temple. This nonverbal cue leads me to consider migraine as a diagnosis. The diagnosis is just the beginning, but finding the trigger that causes the veins of the brain to swell is important to treatment. The real key to treating migraine headaches is to prevent them. Common triggers include fatigue, thunderstorms, insomnia, stress, low blood sugar, pregnancy, ovulation, PMS, and menopause or removal of the ovaries.

If you are over 40, or if your ovaries were removed, testosterone replacement will help prevent headaches from becoming migraines. If your migraines are not completely gone after replacement of testosterone, you should keep a daily journal so that you can identify any nonhormonal triggers that could be causing them. Keep track of when your menstrual cycle begins and ends; what you eat and drink, paying close attention to alcohol, caffeine, and sugar intake; exercise or other physical activities; your sleep habits (quality and quantity); and your energy levels. There are many apps you can use on your smart phone or computer programs to help you quickly and conveniently track these things.

Also note any stressful events or periods of excitement or feeling overwhelmed. It's easy to overlook what may be happening in your life when everything feels chaotic, but these details matter.

THE SECRET FEMALE HORMONE

Once you find your trigger or triggers, you can make lifestyle changes to alleviate your migraines. If the trigger is pollen, thunderstorms, sinus infections, stress, exercise, or allergies, but your migraines began late in your 30s and 40s, the best prevention is to replace testosterone nonorally to determine whether the basic problem is hormonal. If it is, the other triggers will generally not stimulate a headache unless testosterone replacement is halted. If most migraines subside but a few still occur, the most effective prevention includes avoiding red wine, aged cheese, nuts, preservatives, and sugar and taking medications including beta blockers (Inderal or metoprolol) or antidepressants.

Migraines Throughout the Aging Cascade

Migraines triggered by hormonal changes, no matter when they occur, have the same symptoms but differ in the time of life when they begin and the hormones that are responsible for them. Migraines that occur in the premenopausal stage, before age 38, are frequently caused by the hormone estradiol. They typically occur the day before a menstrual period and sometimes on day 14 of the menstrual cycle. Migraines that begin postmenopause and gradually worsen are caused by a lack of testosterone. These generally occur post-TDS and after age 38.

Premenopausal headaches are effectively prevented by shutting down the menstrual cycles with low-dose birth control pills given daily without a break for three months. This decreases the number of headaches to 4 a year instead of 12 and prevents the migraines while the pill is taken. Post-TDS migraine headaches generally begin in our late 30s, and they occur no matter where we are in our menstrual cycle or whether we take birth control pills or not. These migraines do not respond completely to any of the traditional methods of prevention.

Testosterone and Migraines

Current data now indicates that if your testosterone levels are low, you may develop migraine symptoms as an outcome of testosterone deficiency. With testosterone replacement, migraines can disappear.

Recently, research has been done on the use of bio-identical testosterone to stop "cluster migraines"—migraines not easily treated that come in rapid succession over a series of days. This treatment also works for other migraines that occur after age 35, when testosterone typically declines.

The pivotal research on this subject was done by Dr. Mark Stillman of the Neurological Center for Pain at the Cleveland Clinic and published in the January 2006 issue of *Headache*, the journal of the American Headache Society. Dr. Stillman's research demonstrates that the brain's hypothalamus deteriorates as subjects age, and the lack of hypothalamic stimulation of the pituitary and poor response by the testicles and ovaries result in deficient testosterone. One function of the hypothalamus is to chemically stimulate the pituitary gland. When this does not happen, other systems down the line are negatively impacted.

Nonoral bio-identical testosterone stops migraines because it provides free testosterone to cross the blood-brain barrier and enter the brain, where it modulates the hypothalamus and pituitary and adjusts the brain's neurotransmitters. Bio-identical hormone treatment is one of the best migraine treatments available. It works even when patients are told that nothing will work for them.

Migraines were the one symptom Kathy thought would plague her forever. They were also the one symptom she lost immediately after starting postmenopausal replacement with bio-identical testosterone and estradiol pellets. She's been migraine free for ten years and counting, and she wants this success for you as well!

BODY COMPOSITION CHANGES

Women can thank estrogen for their female curves, soft skin, and breasts. But testosterone is also responsible for their youthful female bodies. In fact, women need both hormones in order to have curvy, well-supported, and slender bodies. As long as they produce both hormones in appropriate ratios, they can maintain a healthy-looking body.

The external changes in women's bodies in midlife are the most obvious signs that they are aging and that testosterone has dropped to a critical level. Among the physical changes they see in the mirror with TDS are decreased muscle mass and skin quality and elasticity, increased abdominal fat, cellulite, wrinkles, dry skin, veins, and hair loss.

There are very few women in America who can avoid these physical changes without replacing lost hormones, dieting and exercising to excess, or undergoing plastic surgery. Most women who seek Kathy out feel like they've tried *everything*, and *nothing* has worked.

Dimpled Thighs, Also Called Cellulite!

Women over 40 often complain of "hail damage"—pock marks or dimples on their upper legs, buttocks, hips, and thighs called cellulite. Cellulite is a function of a low-oxygen environment surrounding superficial fat. When testosterone decreases, muscles shrink and do not demand as much oxygen. The fat cells lying on top of those muscles become hypoxic, or "starved" for oxygen, and they succumb to scarring in areas of connective tissue in response. These scars pull the skin down and "dimple" the skin overlying the hypoxic fat.

Treatments for cellulite are aimed at oxygenating the fat, and the best oxygenator is replacing the testosterone so blood and oxygen are drawn to the working and growing muscles. This heals the cellulite from the inside out. For severe cases, or for faster repair, i-Lipo laser or radio wave cellulite treatments help stimulate the blood flow more quickly and help dissolve the fat as well.

Bad Behaviors Contribute to the Body's Decline

When you were younger, you may have been a little reckless with your body. Tanning, drinking alcohol, smoking, and eating unhealthy foods probably didn't affect you the way they do now. There were no visible signs of damage, because you were protected by your body's ability to recover easily in youth. Your abundance of testosterone, estradiol, and growth hormone protected you.

After 40, replacing these missing hormones helps bring your body back to a youthful shape and weight. However, it still requires a healthy lifestyle on your part: the same dose of exercise and healthy eating practices.

Much of what happened to your body is the result of declining levels of free testosterone, estradiol, growth hormone, and possibly thyroid hormone, combined with increased levels of estrone from the adrenal gland. When these changes occur, you become more likely to have serious medical problems such as insulin resistance, which can result in diabetes. This is one of the reasons you need to become much more aware of your carbohydrate consumption after age 40.

When testosterone is present, it sets the stage for the following physical changes:

- Accelerated healing
- Cellulite reduction
- Improved waistline
- Increased blood flow to the skin, muscles, and connective tissue
- Increased dermal (skin) thickness
- Increased lean body mass
- Increased skin moisture and natural oil
- Increased thickness of scalp hair and eyebrows
- Increased volume and definition of muscle and support for the skin layer
- Stimulated collagen production

It remains necessary to maintain a low-carb diet and exercise, and avoid excesses in alcohol consumption. If you do, over a period of about 12 months, these improvements in your body composition help you reacquire a more youthful figure. It takes about a year because your body needs time to restore itself. But if hormone replacement is combined with lifestyle changes, during this time your weight will remain stable (rather than inching upward) as muscle builds and fat decreases. Clothing size and waist measurement will decrease as muscle builds. After a year, weight begins to decrease and continues until you reach your ideal weight. However, damage from the sun and smoking are not reversible in this manner and must be dealt with in other ways.

Restoration of your previous youthful body requires patience, time, work, a low-carb diet, and exercise. Remember: it took years of hormone insufficiency compounded by poor habits to get where you are, and it will take at least a year of testosterone replacement, exercise, and proper diet and nutrition to get back to where you were. But it's easier than you think, especially once you get your energy back. It is truly amazing to watch the reformation of your figure after you have started the journey back to health by restoring your hormone balance to its pre–age 40 levels.

Memory Loss, Cognition, and Testosterone Deprivation

Elaine was starting to feel like she was always forgetting things. "I'm only 50, and sometimes I'll go into a room and can't remember what I was looking for. I have a hard time remembering names, birthdays, directions— things I used to know so well. It seems that it's on the tip of my tongue, but I just can't get it. I'm having some trouble making decisions as well. I'm worried that I may have early-onset Alzheimer's."

Kathy recalls how scared she was after her hysterectomy. She thought maybe they had removed her brain with her uterus and ovaries! First you can't remember a word—then a name. You think it is just a temporary lapse in your recall ability, but it keeps getting worse. In your heart you know there is something wrong, but everyone says you're just "getting older." The catch is that you are in your 40s and still have 40 more years to live! Having a lousy memory for the rest of your life is going to be a terrible journey.

Most of us can't just ignore the fact that we can no longer think clearly because we are older. Our jobs and relationships depend on our ability to think and remember. For most of us, the memory and problem-solving ability are crucial, and we cannot accept the old throwaway, dismissive "It's just aging, so get used to it!"

Vive la Différence

It's important to compare the male and female brains when we talk about memory and cognition problems.

According to an article written several years ago in *Gender Medicine*, women multitask much faster and more effectively than men. This is because they are born with a much larger corpus callosum, the part of the brain that allows communication between both hemispheres (sides of the brain). As a result, their organized left brain talks very effectively—thank you very much—to the emotional and creative right side. This is a good thing, because women were built to do many more things at once than men. Their original roles demanded that they watch children, cook, clean, talk—and switch between all these activities in an instant. These roles have changed, but women's multitasking ability is an asset in the corporate world as well.

Men, on the other hand, have very linear brains. They were designed to hunt, protect, procreate, and work at planting and heavy lifting. Most of us get that, but we need to keep in mind that it is precisely because they *don't* have a developed corpus callosum that they are able to focus so intently on their tasks.

We have recently accepted the fact that at or near age 40 women begin to lose their ability to think in the same way they did when they were younger because their brains' "pacemakers" (pituitary and hypothalamus) begin to slow down at that point, which results in diminished testosterone from the ovary. The research now shows that when testosterone decreases and estradiol increases, neurotransmitters (the chemicals that communicate our thoughts) are decreased. This starts the death of many brain connections, causing loss of memory—including spatial, verbal, and working memory— executive functioning, and attention. Most affected is short-term memory or recall, especially for words. Mood, memory, cognition, behavior, immune function, and balance are also altered. And guess what: menopause makes all these symptoms worse. Women are faced with the potential loss of their organizational skills, ability to multitask, and even the basic ability to think.

Reversing the Decline

This is obviously a problem; everyone needs short- and long-term memory to sustain quality of life. The good news is that simply replacing estradiol and testosterone during the window between a few years premenopause and ten years after menopause can quickly result in regaining memory and thought processes because free testosterone and estradiol cross the blood-brain barrier to increase serotonin and norepinephrine (neurotransmitters), our brain hormones. There's more! A recent study in *Endocrine News* demonstrated that replacement of testosterone that converts to dihydrotestosterone (DHT) restores not just neurotransmitters but synapses and brain cells in mice. That is a whole different level of restoration! It's important to note that estrogen is not enough for most of us; testosterone must also be replaced to restore our memory.

This post-40 mental decline is not Alzheimer's disease or dementia, which many patients say is the disease of which they are most afraid. The genetically predetermined onset of Alzheimer's, however, can be delayed ten years by replacing testosterone prior to menopause. When estradiol is added at menopause, there is an additional ten-year delay in the onset of dementia or Alzheimer's.

Are there specific guidelines to make this work for you? Yes! There are two. First, the two hormones must be replaced in a nonoral form. The subcutaneously inserted hormones (in the form of a bio-identical pellet) cross the blood-brain barrier and increase neurotransmitters better than any other form of bio-identical hormones. Communication among neurons is quickly reestablished. Second, you must not wait more than ten years after TDS begins to replace testosterone, and ten years after menopause to begin the replacement of estrogen!

On average, when Kathy's patients have been treated for one to two months, they are overjoyed with the return of improved mental acuity. They feel their self-worth return, and they no longer suffer the embarrassment of forgetfulness.

In 1997, Lynn had a complete hysterectomy, followed by a bad case of menopause. "I really thought my life was over," she said. "I couldn't sleep, I had terrible headaches, hot flashes, zero energy, and worst of all, I couldn't remember anything. I went to so many doctors who would each treat some of the symptoms, but they never fully understood how bad things were for me . . . I started testosterone therapy and my symptoms began to disappear. I began to feel whole again."

EXERCISE INTOLERANCE

Just when women need exercise in their lives to both calm their brains and tone their bodies, they begin to lose testosterone—and exercise becomes just another chore. Instead of generating energy, exercise zaps it. Women ache and feel drained afterward.

Testosterone is the critical hormone needed to build muscle and decrease fat in the body. It does so by stimulating the pituitary's production of growth hormone that directs muscle to build and strengthen. Testosterone then directs blood flow to muscles and makes them absorb amino acids that allow them to grow. Testosterone also makes muscles clear lactic acid so they don't hurt after exercise.

With high testosterone, muscles are stronger and their endurance for lifting and exercise improves. Additionally, well-testosteronized muscle actually grows to a point where the muscles create heat and burn calories as you sleep. There is no negative impact to the action of testosterone on your muscles and joints. By supplying your body with testosterone, you improve balance, prevent falls, and support running, walking, and maneuvering with your legs, and you prolong your ability to walk and take care of yourself as you age. Blood flow is even increased throughout your body as you use your healthy muscles. Without testosterone you collect lactic acid, the by-product of muscle activity, in your muscles, which causes them to ache long after you exercise. This gives you negative reinforcement to avoid exercise because it hurts.

Phyllis jumped lithely out of bed one morning and stopped abruptly. She turned around and said to her husband, Joe, "I don't hurt all over anymore! I can jump out of bed instead of gradually unfolding as I walk to the bathroom. Wow! Testosterone really works!"

Most women are surprised when they are told that their "arthritis," which occurred about the same time their hormones dropped, will improve with testosterone replacement. Joint aches associated with aging and testosterone are usually related to a loss of synovial fluid, which acts like the oil in your car, lubricating the joints to reduce friction between moving components. With age and loss of testosterone, you lose lubrication, and the friction in the joints wears down cartilage and bone hits bone. The damage done by loss of synovial fluid often necessitates joint replacement. The replacement of testosterone, however, restores the synovial fluid. Joints move freely again without friction, and the procedure can often be delayed, or even avoided.

Sandra was a long-distance runner. At 51, she was still running marathons, but her knees were suddenly hurting and she felt as though they were grinding. She hurt so much that she had to have regular Synvisc injections to increase the synovial fluid in her knees. She was approaching the limit her insurance would spend on this pricey treatment. She had other symptoms of TDS and menopause, but she started testosterone pellets to regain her ability to run. She was surprised that not only could she run marathons again, but the other issues that had started to bother her were also resolved.

As you can see from these two examples, there are two totally different kinds of aches and pains. Sandra's story is about synovial fluids and lubricating them and Phyllis's story is more about the generalized pain reported by many aging women, especially when they awake.

There are, of course, other forms of arthritis and joint pain, but the two types of joint pain—generalized aches and stiffness, and individual pain in certain joints—appear at the same time the other symptoms of testosterone loss occur, and they both improve after adequate levels of testosterone are given in the nonoral form. Improved exercise performance is one of the added benefits of replacing testosterone for patients who are active in sports and exercise.

DRY EYES AND TESTOSTERONE

Dry eye syndrome is very common in women over age 50. While it may not sound like a big deal, tears are necessary for cleaning our eyes, keeping their outer covers moist and hydrated, and protecting the corneas. When we get dry eyes, our tear ducts decrease the production of tears or produce poor quality tears (tears that break down too quickly to be of benefit). Dry eyes can also be caused by loss of oil secretion from the small glands that run along the lash lines. When tears are lacking or of poor quality, the cornea becomes dry, vision is distorted, and the cornea can become scarred.

This condition can prevent you from wearing contacts and cause you to lose vision. Women with dry eyes are often forced to stop wearing contact lenses, just when they need bifocals. In the worst cases of dry eyes, women must wear goggles to prevent evaporation and maintain the moisture in their eyes. They are miserable, and the current treatments rarely cure the problem. Ophthalmologists who refer their patients for testosterone replacement generally continue some of the medications and eye drops. Testosterone eye drops have been evaluated and may be an answer for mild dry eyes, but systemic testosterone is necessary for the worst cases.

Other symptoms of dry eye syndrome include red, scratchy eyes, intolerance to contact lenses, burning and stinging of the eyes, stringy mucous from the eyes, blurred vision, bright rings around oncoming headlights, frequent eye infections, abrasions of the cornea, and poor night vision.

If you think this is a minor problem compared to lost libido and memory loss, think again. The statistics about dry eyes might surprise you. Did you know that 3.2 million American women over 50 suffer from dry eyes? Also, 1.6 million American men over 50 do. Hispanic and Asian women are at a higher risk than other ethnic groups.

Although there are other causes for dry eyes, loss of testosterone is one of the primary ones because every gland that produces "wetness," such as lachrymal ducts (tear ducts), salivary glands, and sweat glands, dry out when the level of testosterone becomes critically low. Decreased testosterone causes increase in cytokines, an inflammatory chemical in blood and tears. Once the lachrymal duct is inflamed, it stops producing tears.

Other Causes of Dry Eyes

There are conditions other than testosterone deprivation that can cause dry eye syndrome, as well:

- Allergies
- Autoimmune disorders such as rheumatoid arthritis, Sjögren's syndrome, and lupus (SLE) Diabetes
- Car air-conditioning ducts
- Contact lenses
- Dry air
- Lasik, blepharoplasty, and other corneal eye surgery
- Medications; e.g., high blood pressure, antihistamines, sleeping pills, some pain relievers
- Pregnancy

Pregnancy is a notable cause of dry eyes. "A significant proportion of women report dry-eye syndrome during pregnancy, especially when they have had at least one prior birth," Joel Schechter, PhD, reported. "Symptoms were four times more likely to be worse during pregnancy than before it. During pregnancy, androgens are deficient, causing insufficient lachrymal gland function."

But pregnancy isn't the only hormonal culprit—there's also menopause. According to an article in *Ob.Gyn. News,* "Dry-eye symptoms occur most frequently in older persons and more often in women than men. The androgens that are released normally by the lachrymal gland help maintain the gland's structural integrity." This substantiates the connection between dry eyes and the endocrine system.

In the worst cases there are generally multiple causes for dry eyes. In these cases testosterone replacement has not been as successful as it is in the patient who presents for some other symptoms of testosterone deprivation syndrome.

Treatment for Dry Eyes

We have noticed for years that patients taking testosterone pellets resolved or improved their problems with dry eyes. Now research has proven that parenteral (intravenous, intramuscular, or pellet) replacement can relieve dry-eye symptoms. Recent findings prove that testosterone is essential to the health of the lachrymal duct and the production of tears.

This connection between testosterone and the resolution of dry-eye syndrome has been discussed and evaluated mostly by ophthalmologists. Because ophthalmologists don't replace hormones, however, they have used topical eye drops compounded with testosterone, but these have been found to be less effective than pellet therapy.

Some ophthalmologists send Kathy their most difficult patients to treat for dry eyes because systemic testosterone—testosterone that is supplied 24/7, such as in pellets—is the best treatment. Many of Kathy's patients have been happily surprised when they could throw away their "cheaters" (over-the-counter reading glasses sold at most drug stores) and put their contacts back in after being treated with testosterone pellets for other reasons.

When Audrey turned 45, her vision began to deteriorate, so like most people, she got contacts. This was a great solution for her because she didn't have to worry about misplacing her glasses. "Not long after, my eyes became too dry to wear contacts," she said. "They scratched me, and I spent a lot of time in the ophthalmologist's office. I started replacing my testosterone for my libido, and voilà, I got my eyes back! I can wear my contacts again. I am so happy!"

Throughout this chapter, we've focused on immediate symptoms of TDS that might be causing you difficulty. It is time to look further to see how the loss of testosterone can impact you as you age. Without testosterone you become susceptible to a host of illnesses commonly associated with being elderly. Many of these conditions are expensive because they restrict your mobility, your ability to live independently, and your ability to function in your daily life. Medicines can be pricey and their side effects problematic, and limitations and discomforts accompany each of these illnesses. On the bright side, most of this can be avoided if you decide to replace your testosterone. In the next chapter, you will learn how this may apply to you.

CHAPTER 6

THE LONG-TERM EFFECTS OF TESTOSTERONE DEFICIENCY

When women consider taking testosterone, they are generally attempting to resolve their immediate symptoms, such as loss of libido, fatigue, or depression. What they don't often think about are the long-term effects of testosterone loss. Part of how you can assess the long-term issues is by examining your inherited risk factors. If you haven't already done so, you need to research your family medical history. By considering the diseases that run in your family tree, you can anticipate what may happen if you do not replace your testosterone. Remember: knowledge is power.

In this chapter, we'll look at all of the potential risks of *not* replacing testosterone.

OSTEOPOROSIS

It is a fact that out of the 10 million people in the U.S. with osteoporosis, 8 million are women! Interestingly, before the advent of a drug to "cure" osteoporosis, doctors rarely attended to the problem. Then, when drugs became available specific to the symptoms of osteoporosis, doctors began to use them. We did not focus on the cause; we just treated the symptom. Now let's work to eliminate the cause of the problem rather than just treat its symptomology. The reason women are so much more likely to develop osteoporosis is that our systems provide us with a tenth of the testosterone men get. When they begin to lose what they have, they are immediately at risk for developing osteoporosis.

The key hormones involved in osteoporosis are testosterone and estradiol. It is interesting that men rarely get the disease unless they are on steroids for asthma or other diseases. The fact is that testosterone makes very thick bones. The female hormone estradiol builds bone, too, but testosterone does it even better.

Bone Construction: How Does It Work?

Bone is made from the building block elements in our diet—the minerals calcium, phosphate, and magnesium. These "blocks" are assembled by using "tools": enzyme systems created from vitamins D and C, which put the blocks together. Vitamin D also helps you absorb calcium from your stomach, and vitamin C provides the "cross-links" to hold the bone together. Bone is not simply constantly building; it is also constantly being broken down. Much like the redecorating we do in our homes, the work is never done!

Hormones are also a factor in bone formation, serving essentially as the project supervisor for bone building. Cortisol and thyroid hormones break down bone; and estradiol, testosterone, parathyroid hormone, and growth hormone build it up. As long as these hormones work in harmony, your bones remain stable and thick. When these building hormones decrease, you reabsorb more bone than you build and your bones get thinner.

What Is Osteoporosis?

Osteoporosis is normally a slow, progressive decrease in bone thickness at the rate of about 1 percent of bone per year. It begins in women before menopause and continues long after. Osteoporosis is serious because it leads to disability, poor posture, chronic pain, broken hips, and crushed vertebrae. Kathy's mother had a severe version of this disease that caused her skeleton to collapse and left her in terrible pain, and she would not wish that on anyone.

Not everyone is at equal risk. As usual, genetics represent the most important risk factor. Generally northern European ancestry is a risk factor and southern European genes are not. The darker your skin, the thicker your bones generally are from birth. After genetics, lifestyle choices and medical treatments also increase your risk of thin bones. Smoking, amphetamine use, Lupron treatment for endometriosis, corticosteroid use, avoiding milk in your diet, lack of sunshine, and a sedentary lifestyle can all lead to thin bones. Some events, like removal of the ovaries, anorexia, or premature menopause, can also cause osteoporosis.

Discovering Osteoporosis: Kathy's Story

When I was 42, my office got a bone density machine. It was very helpful to evaluate our patients and determine who was at risk and who should be treated for bone loss. At the time I had personally undergone three six-month treatments with Lupron to stop chronic pain related to endometriosis and try to achieve another pregnancy. Lupron is an injection that throws a woman into a temporary menopause, with all the symptoms of hormone deprivation.

I had just finished my third round of the drug, checked my bones "for fun," and was stunned to find that I had osteopenia. With this condition, the bones are thin but are not presently at risk of breaking. This is bone loss in the early stages, prior to osteoporosis. With osteoporosis, the bones are so thin that a bone may break during normal activities, and this diagnosis requires intensive treatment.

This came as a complete shock to me, because I have dark skin and eyes, work out regularly, eat dairy products, have never smoked, and was taking no other drugs that would put me at risk. Still, despite all this, I had the very real problem of thin bones. Lupron was the culprit! Three rounds of it had caused my bones to age to those of a 60-year-old—20 years early.

Bisphosphonates (for example, Fosamax) would have been the logical treatment, but they were suspected of making brittle bones. To me, brittle bones are worse than thin bones, so I went without medical treatment awaiting another answer. Two years after my hysterectomy, after treatment with estradiol and testosterone, a routine bone density test revealed that I once again had bones in the normal density range for young, healthy women. I was cured of osteopenia in just two years! I have since seen many of my patients experience the same healthy bone growth with estradiol and testosterone replacement.

Be on the Lookout!

If you do not have osteopenia or osteoporosis yet, you should look for your risk factors in the following symptoms:

- Back pain from nerve compression
- Broken bones in the wrist, foot, rib, or back
- Dowager's hump (hump behind your neck)
- Frequent root canals
- Loss of height
- Spinal stenosis (a narrowing of the open spaces in the spine)

These are all signs of bone loss and impending osteopenia or osteoporosis. Once you know whether you are at risk, then self-evaluate every six months by looking for the presence of these symptoms. Standard of care is that women are given bone density tests at age 50. Our readers may want to seek this earlier or more regularly.

A bone density test films your hips and lower spine. Unlike an X-ray, it involves very low radiation. It takes only a few minutes and is usually administered while you are lying down on a table with your clothes on. The information is processed by a computer and your score is graphed for you to see.

Your bone density score—the most important of which is your T-score—will be in comparison with the bone density of young, healthy women at age 29 and based on the standard deviation (SD) from the mean. If your T-score is within the range of +1 SD to -1 SD, then you are normal. Good for you! If it is more than -1 to -2.5 standard deviations from the mean, you have osteopenia. This result is a warning that if something does not change and your bones continue to decrease yearly by 1 percent per year, osteoporosis is the next step. If your score is over -2.5 SD, then you already have osteoporosis and you are at risk for breaking a bone during normal daily activity.

In the case of bone thickness, just as with the rest of the body, nutrition, exercise, and maintenance hormones are all necessary to stay healthy. All your hormones can be well balanced, but if you don't take in the right building blocks, you can't make healthy bones. If you eat right and take hormones but don't exercise, or if you smoke or take corticosteroids or amphetamines, your bones will still get thin as you age.

To keep bones healthy, every woman should have plenty of calcium in her diet or take a calcium supplement with vitamin D.

The Most Effective Treatments for Osteopenia and Osteoporosis

If you already have osteopenia or osteoporosis, chances are your doctor will recommend some form of bisphosphonate, usually Fosamax, Actonel, or Boniva. Be careful! Recent studies prove that bisphosphonates make bones "look" thick on bone density testing when they are in fact fragile and easily fractured. As a result, Kathy does not recommend this class of drug.

Bisphosphonates have also been accused of causing disintegration of the jawbone. It is not a common side effect but is devastating and disfiguring if you are the one to get it. Other risks of taking those drugs, including muscle pain and esophageal ulcers, make hormone replacement risks look mild. Discuss these risks with your physician. Kathy believes this class of drug would be unnecessary if every woman had her hormones replaced bio-identically.

Everyone who comes to Kathy's office for hormone replacement with testosterone and is already on some form of bisphosphonate is taken off them after one year of treatment. Nothing can compete with the original "bone-builders"—estradiol and testosterone—and with the building blocks of vitamins D and C, calcium, and magnesium.

While studies prove the risks and problems with bisphosphonates, many other studies have proven that estradiol plus testosterone is in fact the very best method to cure osteoporosis. The two hormones together almost double the effect of estradiol alone on bone mass. A study done by J. Studd and M. Savas in 1990 revealed that with estradiol and testosterone pellets, bone density in the spine and hip improved by 8.3 percent at the spine and 2.8 percent at the neck of the femur over a two-year period.

It is also important to remember that the research we are citing is not just gathered from various studies and medical literature but is reconfirmed by the evidence Kathy has seen every day in her medical practice for the last 25 years. Seeing is believing, and medical research is the evidence that proves that what she sees is correct.

Bones are responsive to estrogen and testosterone. With these hormones and an adequate diet, you can protect your bones and yourself from pain, life-threatening fractures, and disability.

Autoimmune Disorders: Rheumatoid Arthritis, SLE (Lupus), Multiple Sclerosis, and Scleroderma

Adult autoimmune disorders can often be prevented by the presence of testosterone in sufficient amounts. For those who have already developed autoimmune disorders, their severity is reduced by the replacement of testosterone.

Let's look at some commonalities among all autoimmune diseases:

- Ages 40 to 60
- Elevated estradiol
- Elevated estrone

- Female
- Genetic risk
- Low testosterone

All autoimmune diseases begin with an infection or exposure to a protein that looks similar to certain tissues in the body. This protein activates the "protective immune response," which increases inflammation and sends out T cells to attack and kill the "foreign" protein. This is a normal response of the body, but in this case it targets the wrong tissue—its own—instead of foreign tissue like bacteria or viruses. This confused response that makes the body attack itself occurs in patients who have a genetic weakness for these diseases and those who are exposed to high-risk viruses.

Demystifying Autoimmune Diseases

T cells and B cells are two types of blood cells called lymphocytes, which are made in the bone marrow. T cells act as killer cells to kill viruses and cancer cells. B cells manufacture antibodies.

There are many types of autoimmune diseases. Medicine divides them according to the tissues the confused antibodies target and the disease's symptoms. Treatment varies by disease, but the one consistent treatment for all autoimmune diseases involves treating with bio-identical testosterone the hormonal imbalance that promotes the destruction of the target tissues.

Hormones can stimulate or modulate the immune system. Estrogen, a stimulator, makes autoimmune diseases worse, while other hormones like testosterone can act as modulators, bringing the system back into the normal range. Other hormonal modulators are prolactin, growth hormone, and vitamin D. Testosterone can suppress immunity when the system is overreacting or stimulate the immune system when it is depressed, as in the case of HIV.

The specifics of the various autoimmune diseases are listed in the following pages. You can see the differences between them, how they present themselves, and how they are treated. Replacing hormones acts as an additional treatment to traditional therapy. Testosterone replacement can be a treatment for these diseases as well as a preventive intervention that will help women avoid auto-immune diseases altogether.

Rheumatoid Arthritis

Rheumatoid arthritis is a result of the body's immune system wrongly attacking joint tissues. If it occurs at the time of meno-pause or premenopause, it can be secondary to a drop in testos-terone. It's more common in women in their 40s than in men at *any* time. Symptoms of rheumatoid arthritis include inflamed, swollen, and painful joints (most specifically knuckles closest to the hand), all fingers pointing toward the little finger, more than one set of joints involved at any one time, generalized inflammation (elevated cardiac CRP blood protein level), and progressive and crippling arthritis.

There are multiple causes of rheumatoid arthritis. It might be triggered by a hypersensitive immune system or a family history of other autoimmune diseases, such as lupus, thyroiditis, or Sjögren's syndrome.

Traditional therapy for rheumatoid arthritis has been non-steroidal anti-inflammatory drugs (NSAID) like Motrin, Relafen, or Aleve, as well as steroids such as prednisone. More recently, sufferers have undergone "gold therapy" or Enbrel intravenous ther-apy. These traditional treatments come with their own side effects. NSAIDs carry the risk of ulcers and bleeding; steroids and Enbrel suppress your immune system, opening you up to many bacteria, viruses, and cancers; and gold therapy places your kidneys at risk.

The newest research on rheumatoid arthritis has demonstrated that testosterone deprivation between ages 40 and 50 is often a trigger. Treatment with bio-identical testosterone and Arimidex, which blocks the production of estrone, stops the progression of the joint changes and balances the immune system. Moreover, testosterone increases synovial fluid in the joints and modulates the immune system.

In addition to testosterone pellet treatment, other nontraditional therapies have included bio-identical hormone replacement therapy (*non*pellet HRT), nutritional therapy, chelation therapy, and acupuncture. In Chapter 9, you'll learn more about these different methods of hormone replacement.

If you have been successfully treated for rheumatoid arthritis in a traditional fashion, that is great! If you haven't found relief, try balancing your hormones. We have treated many rheumatoid arthritis sufferers and have found that testosterone is the key: it increases the normal joint fluid and decreases inflammation.

Systemic Lupus Erythematosus (SLE) or Lupus

Annie was in her late 30s when she began to lose her eyesight. She had a rare form of SLE that attacks the retina and progressively decreases sight. She found amazing specialists who treated her with every possible method for her illness. Because SLE is an autoimmune disease that destroys tissue through a hyperactive immune system, Annie was given high-dose steroids to stop the disease.

Over the course of her treatment, Annie gained 60 pounds. This is common among women who take steroids for any condition, but Annie was no less upset. She also had to have monthly eye injections, but blindness still progressed.

Annie came to Kathy to see if hormone therapy would help her lose weight and regain her sex drive. To her surprise, testosterone not only helped with her weight loss and libido—it stopped the progression of her blindness. She no longer had to have shots in her eye. She continued her other medications for lupus, but her sight did not deteriorate one bit further!

Lupus is an autoimmune disease that is 12 times more common in women than in men. There is also a difference in occurrence based on race. Women of African descent have the highest rate of SLE, followed by Asian women and then Caucasian women. Where we live also affects our chance of getting the disease. There are about 54 new cases of SLE per 100,000 in the U.S. per year, but Great Britain has a lower incidence of SLE, at 28 new cases per 100,000.

Genetics play a part in our risk of lupus, but our environment is also a factor. Studies show that exposure to certain drugs as well as viruses can increase the risk of getting the disease.

The symptoms of this disease and the tests used to identify it are different from other autoimmune diseases. Lupus anti-bodies attack the skin, heart pericardium, lungs, kidneys, eyes, nerves, and blood vessels. The symptoms associated with lupus include arthritis; red rash across the cheeks (shaped like a butter-fly); myocarditis, pericarditis, and pleurisy (inflammation of the heart muscle, the sack around the heart, and the thin covering around the lungs); nephritis—inflammation of the kidneys caus-ing blood in the urine and damage to the kidneys; Raynaud's phenomenon (transient red, white, and blue hands that are pain-ful); and seizures.

Scleroderma

This autoimmune disease begins with fatigue, muscle pain, swelling of the hands, and Raynaud's phenomenon. It occurs five times as often in women as in men. It is also more common in the U.S. than in Britain and the rest of Europe. Scleroderma does its damage by attacking the blood. This causes fibrosis and scar tissue in all the vessels, even small ones. The vessels develop so much fibrosis that no blood can get through. The digits, fingers, and toes are subsequently damaged because the fibrosis cuts off the blood supply.

The symptoms of scleroderma include:

- Broken blood vessels on the palm of the hand
- Dry mouth, eyes, and vagina
- Fatigue

- Necrosis of the fingers
- Pepper and salt skin pigmentation
- Poor motility of the esophagus, causing food to stick in the middle of the esophagus
- Pulmonary fibrosis—"honeycomb lung"
- Shiny fingertips
- Skin thickening

Testing for this autoimmune disease is more difficult than some of the others, and some sufferers have no positive tests at all. The few tests that are positive in small percentages of the patients who have scleroderma include these:

- ANA, which detects antinuclear antibodies
- Antitopoisomerase antibody, anti-RNA polymerase III antibody, and anticentromere antibody

This diagnosis is not one to be taken lightly; however, scleroderma is a relatively rare disease.

Many sufferers discover that it generally responds well to testosterone replacement and Arimidex to decrease estrone levels. This positive response is due to testosterone's effect on inflammation. Testosterone decreases the scarring by decreasing the inflammation in the vessels.

Multiple Sclerosis

Most women who live in the northern U.S. have at least one friend with this progressive and debilitating disease. Doctors have recently begun to consider MS an autoimmune disease, triggered by a viral infection in women with a genetic weakness that allows the body to attack the myelin sheath that "insulates" all of our nerves. The final result can be paraplegia or quadriplegia, and sometimes even death. Thankfully, testosterone replacement has been found to stop the progression of this debilitating disease.

Symptoms of MS include recurrent, progressive loss of muscle tone, loss of balance, loss of vision or voice, severe pain and spastic muscle movements, loss of bladder and bowel control, decrease in muscle strength, and loss of sight from attacks on the optic nerve.

Diagnosis of MS is made by a physical exam including blood tests, a history of recurrent symptoms, and an MRI of the brain and spine.

After years of study, it has been determined that any treatment that decreases the immune system or modulates it tends to slow the progression of symptoms. Traditional medications include interferon and immunosuppressive medications. Testosterone is key to giving a woman with MS the best chance to respond to other medications. We have found that MS stops progressing or remains in remission with testosterone replacement. Testosterone pellets have no adverse side effects other than facial hair—well worth it when you can heal a devastating illness like MS.

Denise was 42 when she was diagnosed with MS. She had been a very energetic woman, caring for three children, writing music, singing, and playing the guitar—and, of course, dancing. Over the next three years her ability to fully engage in her favorite physical activities had disappeared. She reluctantly started testosterone replacement with pellets when she had no other therapies to try. By now she had been let down by so many treatments that she had become a skeptic.

Six weeks after starting testosterone pellets she noticed the pain was diminishing. She was back on her feet, chasing after the kids and dancing with her husband in the kitchen. With only one dose of testosterone, she was slowly transformed back into the lovely, positive, and energetic person she had been before MS!

As a physician, Kathy has always felt helpless with this disease because it seemed to randomly select victims in their prime. Testosterone treatment gave us a powerful weapon to fight the progression of MS. It is important to remember that patients should not abandon traditional medications necessary to fight this disease.

Testosterone should be added to the treatment plan and is not a substitute for other medications.

CHRONIC FATIGUE SYNDROME AND FIBROMYALGIA

Chronic fatigue syndrome (CFS) is a common yet relatively new illness. It has only been recognized as a true physical illness in the last 15 years. Medical doctors don't usually take it seriously, and as a result patients with this illness are often left with a poor quality of life.

A patient is considered to have CFS if they have four or more of the following symptoms:

- Decreased ability to think
- Depression
- Multiple joint pain
- Muscle pain
- New headaches
- Nonrefreshing sleep
- Postexertional malaise
- Severe, incapacitating fatigue
- Short-term memory loss
- Sleep disturbance
- Sore throat
- Tender cervical or axillary lymph nodes

CFS is often confused by both doctors and patients with fibromyalgia because both diseases have the same initial symptoms of fatigue and generalized aching, yet the diseases have different causes. CFS is caused by an ongoing infection that is impossible to eradicate because the immune system has become overwhelmed and can no longer kill the infection. In contrast, fibromyalgia may be a type of autoimmune disease but medicine has not yet categorized it as such.

A Closer Look at Chronic Fatigue Syndrome

The causes of CFS include viruses and bacteria that people commonly get and fight successfully, healing quickly and without residual issues. In the case of CFS, however, the patient cannot overcome the infection and suffers with it for a long period of time. It can also be caused by an old virus that has never been fully suppressed and reemerges. All of these causes make chronic fatigue a frustrating and debilitating illness.

Causes of CFS
Viruses
• CMV—cyclomegalovirus • Epstein-Barr virus (EBV)—the cause of mononucleosis • Human Herpes virus (HHV-6)—resistant to the drug acyclovir
Bacteria
• Chlamydia • Lyme disease • Mycoplasma
Generally the most common virus causing this disease is the Epstein-Barr virus (mononucleosis). CFS caused by viruses is the hardest to treat because there are few potent antivirals available.

Testing for CFS

You can take clinical tests to diagnose CFS. Ask your doctor to help you determine which, if any, you might need to determine whether you have chronic fatigue syndrome.

- Blood pressure—orthostatic hypotension
- BUN, creatinine, ALT, AST
- CBC (blood count) with differential
- Cortisol, ACTH, CRH (all low)
- Cytokines and inflammation (increased)
- +EBNa for EBV (mono)
- Lipids (high cholesterol)
- Liver enzymes (high alkaline phosphatase, low LDH)
- Lyme disease titers
- MRI—decreased perfusion of the brain
- Parvovirus, influenza, enterovirus
- Select TORCH titers (toxoplasmosis/CMV/H herpes virus-6 IgG)

Treatment Options for CFS

CFS can be treated in two general ways: kill the infecting organism or improve the function of the immune system so the body can rid itself of the infection.

There is specific treatment for the EBV (Epstein-Barr) and CMV (cytomegalovirus) viruses, which cause CFS. Research was done by Dr. Jose Montoya at Stanford University, who found that these viruses respond to the antiviral drug Valcyte. It is approved by the FDA only for patients with AIDS and one of these viruses; however, it works very well for CFS.

Other treatments for CFS, such as vitamins and dietary restrictions, are supportive. In terms of CFS previously treated with measures like rest, vitamins, and nutrition, the next step is to replace what placed the patient at risk for the infection in the beginning: a suppressed immune system caused by a natural loss of testosterone. CFS patients require a higher dose of testosterone to resolve their symptoms than the uncomplicated patient with TDS, but most of the time, testosterone improves symptoms, if not the infection itself.

Treatment for Chronic Fatigue

Diet Restriction

Alcohol

Caffeine

Sugar

Vitamin K

White flour and other processed carbs

Vitamins

Vemma nutritional supplement, 2 doses/day

Other liquid or chewable nutritional supplement derived from whole grain foods

And/or all of the following

Vitamin C 1,000 mg/day

Vitamin E 800 MIU/day

Beta-carotene (vitamin A) 3,500 mg/day

Bioflavinoids (from citrus rind) 500 mg/day

B1=thiamine (brain functioning) 75 mg/day

B2=riboflavin 475 mg/day → energy

B3=niacin 50 mg/day → heart health, dopamine, memory

Pantothenic acid 50 mg/day → adrenal gland function

B6=pyridoxine 85 mg/day (CF 250 mg/day) → improves immune function, thyroid function, and fluid retention

B12=Sublingual tablet or drops or im shot (1,000 mcg/day or 10,000 mcg q 10 days im) → relieves joint pain, aches, memory loss, fatigue; removes toxins like nitric oxide, depression

Folic acid 800 mcg/day → prevents dementia; helps memory and immune function

Biotin 200 mcg/day → enzyme cofactor for hair loss and brain function

Vitamin D3 (1–4,000 IU/day) → immune function

Amino Acids
Serine 500–1,000/day for immune function
Arginine 200 mg/day → growth hormone, but also increases nitric acid—use carefully
Methionine 100–300 mg/day (part of Sam-e)—keeps levels low
NAC 250–650 mg/day → Glutathione → healing and immune function

Hormones
Testosterone given with pellets achieving a moderately high dose
Replace cortisol if low
Replace thyroid hormone if low
Suppress elevated prolactin with Dostinex or Pariodel

Note: im stands for intramuscular.

Testosterone deprivation can cause CFS, since it is commonly the reason the immune system crashed to begin with.

Fibromyalgia

Unlike CFS, fibromyalgia is not well understood. The experts consider it a possible autoimmune disease or a disordered pain perception syndrome. The patients who have been diagnosed with this illness come to Kathy's office have had their lives drastically affected by this illness. The primary symptom is muscular pain that is incapacitating. It responds to testosterone treatment and is often accompanied by a diagnosis of CFS.

Patients are considered to have fibromyalgia if they have the following symptoms:

- Fatigue
- More than 11 defined tender points in soft tissue (not joints)
- Nonrefreshing sleep
- Stiffness

This illness is more common in women than in men, and like most autoimmune diseases, it follows genetic family groups and usually follows a traumatic event such as physical injury, infection, or hospital admission. Fibromyalgia causes insomnia and is often treated by mainstream medicine with amitriptyline, an antidepressant, which improves symptoms of pain and insomnia. Pain medications, acupuncture, and rest are currently recommended for fibromyalgia patients, but rarely is testosterone considered. When fibromyalgia is treated with bio-identical testosterone, symptoms frequently stop, and then other medications are not necessary.

Both CFS and fibromyalgia result from an abnormality of the immune system. Chronic fatigue is from a depressed immune system, and fibromyalgia is most likely from an overactive, misdirected one.

Testosterone impacts the immune system in a variety of ways. When testosterone decreases, the number and activity of T cells decrease and patients are much more susceptible to both viruses and bacteria, as well as cancer cells.

There are life events that suppress the immune system and place a woman at risk for getting CFS or fibromyalgia, including severe and long-lasting stress, other chronic illnesses that suppress the immune system, chemotherapy, and genetic immune suppression.

The Immune System and Aging

The progressive decline in hormones as we age is thought to result in impaired immunity. This not only causes an increase in autoimmune disease but is also the cause of the increase in cancers as we age. An intact immune system prevents the cells that continually become precancer cells from growing. Our immune system hunts down abnormal cells and kills them. If the system is down, we are unprotected from abnormal cells growing and becoming cancer. It is certainly a complicated process, but the takeaway is that the diseases of aging that we most fear are often prevented by restoring normal levels of hormones and a normal immune system.

Dementia, Alzheimer's Disease and Parkinson's Disease

Kelly, a 43-year-old teacher, came to see Kathy because she was experiencing some short-term focusing problems. She had the sense that she could not remember anything for more than ten minutes and was nervous that this would affect her job performance. She also shared that both of her parents, now in their 70s, were suffering from Alzheimer's. Kelly was terrified that she was developing this disease, too. We were able to reassure her that by replacing her lost testosterone, we could alleviate her other symptoms and fix her recall problems.

Dementia

Most of us know that the diagnosis of dementia is serious and generally associated with old age or a head injury. It is particularly devastating when it occurs in youthful, productive women under the age of 70.

Dementia is an "umbrella term" that encompasses many types of conditions that have cognitive defects, or, in simpler terms, the inability to think, as the primary symptom. The fact that dementia affects 35.6 million people worldwide—a number that is increasing as our life expectancy soars—is worrisome, but the *most* worrisome aspect of dementia is when it is given to you as *your* diagnosis!

We wrote this section to inform patients and their families that "it ain't over till it's over" and that a simple thing like testosterone pellets can stop most dementia and Alzheimer's disease dead in their progressive tracks.

The Nature and Causes of Dementia

Dementia generally starts with the inability to recall people's names or the word for certain items. This is usually followed by an inability to remember recent events, which then progresses to an inability to remember events from the more distant past. While we all recognize these symptoms, which are the result of deterioration of the neurons—or the electric wiring of our brains—as associated with old age, the loss of word recognition, problem solving, and memory is different in each individual. I think viewing this condition as a short circuit in our brains is the best way for a layperson to understand the problem.

Many things can trigger dementia. Strokes, which are caused by vascular malfunction, are one of the most common because they can damage areas in the brain. One cause of stroke is a clot that blocks the blood vessel and prevents blood flow. Also, as we get older our blood vessels narrow and weaken. Blood vessels become more susceptible to rupture, which can result from high blood pressure, or an abnormal or weak vessel leaks blood into the brain. Both blockage and rupture can cause the permanent death of parts of the brain. When this brain damage affects thought, it is called "vascular dementia." Permanent brain damage from a stroke leaves the patient with deficits in his or her ability to think, move, or feel.

Good nutrition, low inflammation, normal cholesterol, normal blood pressure, and exercise all help to prevent strokes and the other changes associated with aging. The most important factor in preventing stroke and the damages of aging, however, may be the replacement of all hormones that decrease with age: estradiol, testosterone, growth hormone, thyroid hormone, and corticosteroids. Without the replacement of estradiol and testosterone, our brains are more sensitive to the effects of low oxygen and are more likely to be lined with cholesterol plaque. This is one of the reasons dementia from strokes is more common in older patients.

Dementia can also be caused by traumatic head injury. These can be repetitive, such as those suffered during competitive contact sports, or from a single incident such as an auto accident. In these situations dementia may not even show up immediately because the real injury is often to the pituitary gland. When injured, the pituitary stops secreting growth hormone and/or stimulating all the usual hormone secretions from the ovaries, thyroid, or adrenals. The onset of dementia is delayed because this drop in production is not immediate, but eventually it not only makes the patient feel much older but also slowly accelerates aging. The brain fails to repair itself and so collects plaque and loses neurotransmitters. The outcome is the loss of effective memory and problem-solving ability.

Head injuries in athletes and auto-accident victims represent a relatively new area of study for endocrinologists and neurologists. The National Football League has become increasingly aware of the potential long-term effects of repetitive concussion, but the same injuries have not yet been studied in female athletes. The current expert on this subject is Dr. Mark Gordon, medical director of Millennium Health Centers in Southern California, who has just released a book for doctors called *The Clinical Application of Interventional Endocrinology*. It features an entire chapter on the outcome of head injury in athletics and includes a discussion of hormone replacement as a recommended treatment.

How Do Hormones Prevent the Progression of Dementia?

Estradiol and testosterone prevent dementia by several mechanisms. They repair neurons in the brain and prevent death of neurons, increase production of neurotransmitters, decrease inflammation, decrease shrinkage of the brain after menopause, increase blood flow and oxygen to the brain through dilation of blood vessels, and increase the use of glucose improving thought processes and speed of thought.

Specifically, if women's testosterone and estrogen levels do not remain in the young, healthy range, their brains begin to shrink and their neurons die and don't replace themselves. This causes a loss of the ability to think, remember, and solve problems. When the process devolves to a certain point, we are no longer able to care for ourselves. This is a quality-of-life issue, as well as a practical problem for women and their families. This part of aging is the most obvious motivator for replacing estradiol and testosterone for women who want to remain independent.

Timing is everything when we consider replacement of hormones. There is a ten-year window after your hormones drop below young, healthy levels during which you can replace them and maintain your brain size and function. Replacing estradiol and testosterone within this window delays the onset of all types of dementia by ten years for each hormone replaced. If you want to prevent dementia, then replacing both hormones will effectively delay the onset of dementia by 20 years! Brain cells are irretrievable beyond this window of opportunity.

Longer lives mean more years lived after TDS and menopause, which means the rate of Alzheimer's disease in women will increase. The newest research—including the Multi-Institutional Research in Alzheimer's Genetic Epidemiology study and the Women's Health Initiative Memory Study—report the finding that this ten-year testosterone-replacement window specifically prevents and/or delays the onset of Alzheimer's. This is also true of other neurological diseases related to aging and testosterone depletion, including Parkinson's, dementia secondary to toxins, strokes, trauma, and other circulation deficits. Analysis by the Mayo Clinic Cohort Study of Oophorectomy and Aging found that if bilateral removal of the ovaries occurred without estrogen replacement, there was an increased risk of Parkinson's disease, cognitive impairment, dementia, anxiety, and depression.

A 2002 article in the *Journal of the American Medical Association* also showed that some serious cognitive diseases can be delayed through the use of estradiol and testosterone therapy. The protective mechanism for estradiol is antioxidant action on the neurons of the brain, which prevents the accumulation of amyloid, a corrosive material that coats the neurons and causes Alzheimer's disease. Estrogen replacement works to prevent this corrosive impact in the brain.

There is sufficient scientific evidence that replacement of estradiol and testosterone *prevents* dementia and Alzheimer's disease, but there is currently no evidence that replacement can reverse or halt the progression of the disease. Even though Kathy has personally been successful in reversing the mental changes in women who have early-onset dementia of many types, further studies must be undertaken to prove that what she sees every day is repeatable.

Alzheimer's Disease

Alzheimer's disease is a particular type of dementia that is genetic rather than being caused by an injury or stroke. It affected 13.7 million people in 2011. No matter how many women are doomed to get this disease, all it takes is one if that one is you!

If a patient has Alzheimer's, Parkinson's, or early-onset dementia, it may be preventable through bio-identical hormone replacement. Habib Rehman in *Gender Medicine* describes how your natural hormones, at premenopausal levels, protect you from brain degeneration. After menopause, you experience low levels of estradiol and testosterone and increased levels of LH (luteinizing hormone) and FSH (follicle-stimulating hormone), your pituitary hormones essential for reproduction. In response to these increased levels, you make decreased levels of the hormone inhibin, which causes the neurons of the brain to degenerate. The key is to use enough bio-identical hormones to suppress FSH and LH, which in turn prevents Alzheimer's.

We can suppress FSH/LH below menopausal levels by giving generous doses of estradiol and testosterone. This is in direct opposition to the guidelines by the American Congress of Obstetricians and Gynecology (ACOG), which recommends all doctors give the lowest possible dose of estradiol replacement for postmenopausal women—and does not mention testosterone at all. If that guideline is followed by thousands of American OB/GYNs, millions of women will be misled into a life with a high risk for dementia.

Of course, Alzheimer's disease is more common in people who have the gene for it and who have early menopause and testosterone deprivation without hormone replacement. The onset of Alzheimer's disease generally occurs between the ages of 60 and 75, and earlier in women than in men. Alzheimer's is diagnosed by a CT or MRI scan of the brain that shows a characteristic shrinkage of the brain resulting from neuron (brain cell) death, following plaques that form on the neurons and choke them to an early death.

In 2002, P. P. Zandi studied a group of older men and women in Cache County, Utah, and compared the rate of Alzheimer's between men and women, as well as between women who did not take hormone replacement therapy (HRT) and women who did take HRT. He found that women had almost double the rate of Alzheimer's disease when compared with men if they did not take HRT.

When the investigators from Johns Hopkins compared women who did not take HRT with those who did, they found that women without HRT had at least double the rate of Alzheimer's disease compared to the women who did take HRT. If women took HRT for ten years or more, they had the same risk as men, which was much lower.

This study concluded that HRT users had a reduced risk of Alzheimer's disease, and the longer it was used the lower the risk, with the lowest rate found in women who took HRT for ten years or more.

Parkinson's Disease

Parkinson's disease affects more than 1 percent of Americans over 65 and is generally seen more in men than in women. Parkinson's has been linked to both genetic and environmental causes, as well as the loss of testosterone. It can be modulated by testosterone and estradiol, in addition to other drugs specific to increasing the production of dopamine, a neurotransmitter that is depleted in Parkinson's patients as a result of damage to the neurons that produce it. While the average age of onset of Parkinson's is around

60, the neuronal damage is believed to begin seven to ten years before the initial symptoms.

The list of symptoms associated with Parkinson's disease is long and varied and can include:

- Constipation
- Decreased ability to function socially
- Difficulty keeping balance
- Difficulty swallowing
- Fatigue
- Loss of facial expression
- Memory and cognitive difficulty
- Mood changes; depression/anxiety; apathy
- Slow, plodding movement; stiffness; weakness
- Speech changes
- Tremors

Parkinson's disease is also associated with early menopause or hysterectomy with removal of ovaries in women. It occurs more often in women who do not take hormone replacement therapy after menopause. (It occurs in men at a later average age, after andropause.) Estradiol stimulates dopamine release and in doing so enhances the brain's electrical and chemical communication. Estradiol has been used as a staple in nursing homes to decrease dementia in general and specifically Parkinson's disease in women.

Estradiol acts as an antioxidant and repairs damaged cells that make dopamine by supporting the growth of new neurons. Testosterone replacement in men is very effective in slowing the progression of the symptoms of Parkinson's disease and can often cause some symptoms to regress to normal. Testosterone is most effective on the symptoms of memory loss, proprioception and balance, attention, and fine motor coordination.

The proven ability of bio-identical hormone replacement to forestall or entirely prevent the onset of Alzheimer's and dementia is often obscured by the hoopla generated by pharmaceutical companies over new medicines they have produced to treat these diseases (and to realize far more profit than can be made with bio-identical hormones). Kathy generally tells her patients who already have Alzheimer's disease that they should take the prescribed medications and replace estradiol and testosterone to give them the best chance of stopping this devastating illness. And again, subdermal pellets are by far the *most* effective delivery system for these hormones, for the reasons previously stated. Be sure to check out Chapter 9 to learn more about why this is so.

Understanding the importance of both estradiol and testosterone is critical for the prevention and treatment of the widespread debilitating diseases that make up the larger diagnosis of dementia, for which the incidence rate is increasing every year. We know we can slow it down in this generation and stop it in the next through preventive replacement after age 40 of estradiol and testosterone in a bio-identical pellet delivery system for everyone with risk factors. This should be encouraging to those of us who watched our parents and grandparents lose themselves, body and soul, to diseases that were once thought hopeless. If we can convince the medical community to center on prevention and replacement rather than playing catch-up using imperfect medications, it seems we have a chance!

SARCOPENIA

Jane's mother, Evelyn, is 75 years old and sharp as a tack, but she looks very old. Her thin, bent posture tells the story of her minimal muscle mass, and she shuffles as she walks behind her walker. Evelyn has pain in all of her limbs, which makes her irritable. Her muscle loss is most evident in her calves and arms, where her skin literally hangs off her bones. Evelyn's body has deteriorated to the point where she can no longer live on her own. Jane is worried about her mother and concerned that she'll suffer the same fate in 25 years.

Sarcopenia is the degenerative loss of muscle mass leading to frailty and, often, assisted living. It's a difficult subject for anyone who is currently intact, mobile, and independent to think about. But for many, it is the inevitable end result of aging without replacement of testosterone. Most women are the caretakers of their families, and they need their independence and a well-functioning body to accomplish their tasks. Sarcopenia eventually advances to a point where women cannot walk, run, lift, drive, or push. It leads them to the unthinkable end of their productive lives.

Even though you may consider this situation to be far in the future, you must think about it now, because loss of muscle and strength begins in the 40s and 50s and requires treatment long before you have any signs of frailty. Testosterone replacement is the only treatment available for the majority of people to prevent frailty and sarcopenia. Replacing testosterone in midlife is somewhat like making an investment so you don't require long-term-care insurance for a future life in a nursing home.

Coming Face-to-Face with Sarcopenia: Kathy's Experience

Like Jane and many of my patients, I started caring for an elderly parent, in my case my mother. Her experience followed the time line I described, with frailty being the final blow. She never expected to live as long as she did (into her 90s), and it was difficult to watch as her body withered away.

Following my mother's journey inspired me to investigate what I could do to avoid the same disintegration of muscles, bones, and mind, and to ensure that I can be independent for as long as I live. In the process I discovered two things: life should be lived as if we will live for a long time, saving our bodies' liveliness just like we save our money to support us for the long run; and replacing testosterone—and preferably all of our missing hormones (estrogen, thyroid hormone, and possibly growth hormone) is the only way I have found that will protect us from the disabling frailty so many of our mothers experienced in their final years.

What Causes Sarcopenia?

Until recently medicine did not connect the dots between the cause and effect of testosterone loss, the high number of women in nursing homes, and the high and rising cost of medical care in the U.S. In the last ten years, however, sarcopenia's devastating economic impact has brought this issue to the forefront of politics and budgeting for Medicare.

The aging cascade leading to frailty seems to begin when we lose muscle and subsequently lose our balance, leading to a fall. Our muscles support our balance and when they degenerate, we need to do something to restore them. Without testosterone replacement, women fall, and often brittle bones break, sending them to a rehab or nursing facility to learn how to walk again. We explained earlier how testosterone operates to help restore muscle mass and strength. Now we are discussing its impact on the density and strength of the bones. During their recovery time, the frailest are not able to regain their muscle strength and often succumb to blood clots or pneumonia, which often lead to death.

Looking at this process as a whole, it's pretty clear that the origin of sarcopenia is not the fall itself but the loss of balance from the decreased muscle mass resulting from years of untreated testosterone deficiency.

Sarcopenia Exposed

Frailty and sarcopenia share a variety of symptoms, but they are actually different. Frailty is associated with weight loss, mostly muscle loss replaced with fat; weakness; slow walking speed; exhaustion; and decreased physical activity. Sarcopenia, on the other hand, has the following attributes: sagging muscles on arms and legs; posture that leans forward, with the gaze toward the floor; loss of mass in shoulders and hips with a distended abdomen; poor balance, expressed with hesitance in walking or climbing stairs or the inability to rise out of a chair; shaky hands; and slowness of thought. Sarcopenia is often the precursor to the frailty of old age.

Most of us remember our grandparents, and possibly our parents, with some of these symptoms. Kathy remembers both of her parents turning the corner into the bodily appearance that heralded their loss of independence. Her mother always walked fast and had good posture. She could always keep up with Kathy. In her last few years, she lost muscle mass, bent over, and became unsure of her balance. She began to hold on to Kathy and kept her head down looking at the ground. Kathy's father was a tennis player and runner, but she began to see the same physical symptoms in him when he turned 80. The physical changes aren't just about muscles and posture; these signs are the visible changes. As usual, what goes on behind the scenes in the aging of our bodies all comes back to how the body responds to losing the one essential hormone: testosterone.

Why Testosterone Loss Causes Muscle Loss and Frailty

Many scientists are embroiled in studying microscopic chemical changes in the body that are associated with aging. Rarely do they relate those findings to one hormone, bodily secretion, human activity, or habit that actually is the trigger for those minute chemical changes.

Their myopic view causes them to miss the big picture; the decrease in testosterone in our 40s and 50s represents the first hormone to fall in the aging cascade. The first change in aging is inflammation. Testosterone is an anti-inflammatory hormone, and its loss triggers inflammation of all of our tissues. Inflammation is destructive when it is a constant condition. Inflammation causes high blood pressure, heart disease, stroke, arthritis, and muscle pain. It is a pivotal catalyst to what ages and eventually kills us.

The role of the loss of testosterone in aging does not stop with the initiation of inflammation. Loss of testosterone causes muscles to shrink and bones to dissolve by diverting blood flow and therefore halting anabolic growth and repair of muscles. The loss of muscle then causes a direct effect on the brain by secreting a substance that makes cerebral blood vessels contract and deliver less oxygen to the brain. In short, without muscles you literally lose your ability to think! This makes exercise in your youth and middle age look much more important, doesn't it?

Conquering Sarcopenia and Frailty with Testosterone—at 85!

One older couple in Kathy's practice illustrates the amazing restorative benefits of testosterone even after the age of 80.

Rita started taking testosterone pellets in addition to estradiol pellets in her 70s. Over the years, she seemed to age less than her friends. In fact, they started calling her a "vampire" because she looked and acted like she was 20 years younger than everyone else.

Rita's husband, Ed, was a very busy and productive man who didn't seem to slow down until he was 85. At that point he had to undergo his second joint replacement. Unlike what followed his previous surgery a few years earlier, he was unable to regain his ability to walk. Ed managed multiple real-estate properties himself, fixed roofs and plumbing, and was accustomed to an active life. Loss of mobility was not acceptable for him.

The debilitation that followed Ed's second surgery brought on a deep depression. No matter how much physical therapy he tried, he could not stand up. In desperation, Rita asked Kathy if it would be possible for Ed to try testosterone pellet replacement, too. Kathy prefers to start replacement of testosterone in both men and women before 75, as the side effects are less common. After an evaluation, however, she acquiesced.

She's glad she did! Ed had an amazing experience using testosterone to conquer his frailty. Within a month, he graduated from a wheelchair to a walker, and then to a cane. The second month, he was back to maintaining all of his properties, as independent as ever with one great exception—he also had a great sex drive and performance! That was years ago, and he is going strong to this day! He is muscled, balanced, strong, and certainly no longer frail.

No one wants to live forever, but Ed and Rita are enjoying their golden years, living well and independently.

Loss of movement related to diminished testosterone represents yet another process in the aging cascade. When we stop moving because we are frail and we ache, other conditions result from our immobility. Our veins clog with blood and we get clots, bone mar-row ceases to make blood cells that deliver oxygen, nerves and muscles stop communicating, and weakness increases. Our bones require muscles and movement to stay thick, and strong bones become osteoporotic with weak muscles. The immune system and immune globulins from the thymus stop production. This process signals the end of life, and poor movement multiplies the symp-toms by discouraging further movement.

By this point I hope you are motivated to rethink aging and become older in a different fashion than your parents and grand-parents did! Unlike them, you have higher stakes because you will be old for a longer period of time. Who among us wants to live in a nursing home or depend on our children when we could prevent this easily and effectively?

INSULIN RESISTANCE, TYPE 2 DIABETES, AND OBESITY

Andrea was 45 when she realized she had to make a change. She was fatigued, gaining weight, and unable to sleep. She went to her primary-care doctor, who told her she had prediabetes, and if she didn't lose weight, pretty soon she'd have type 2 diabetes. But he didn't tell her how to lose weight, and he wouldn't give her medicine unless she had diabetes. Andrea was shocked. When her friend Beth told her about her hormone specialist, she decided she would see one, too. She was given replacement testosterone, but she was not menopausal yet so did not need estrogen. Andrea was also placed on Victoza and a diet and exercise program. Four months later her weight was down 20 pounds. She was exercising and feeling great! Andrea didn't sit around and wait for the storm of diabetes to knock her down—she got help!

Type 2 diabetes, or diabetes that is associated with obesity, is fast becoming medicine's number one enemy! The disease itself affects a third of Americans, and the majority of all medical research dollars are spent on strategies for treating and preventing it.

Diabetes is so important because it affects every cell in the body and leads to devastating medical consequences. It is Kathy's belief that we must reverse the current trend toward diabetes instead of just accepting our fate. That, of course, is one of the themes of this book! We can still intervene during the stage known as prediabetes to prevent and avoid further development of this deadly illness. We need to learn to treat it in ways that allow us to avoid the inevitable diseases that follow.

Testosterone replacement is one of the keys to blocking the onset of diabetes or reversing its progression if it is already present. Doesn't it make more sense to use one hormone to prevent dozens of symptoms and the debilitating diseases that follow rather than try to play catch-up?

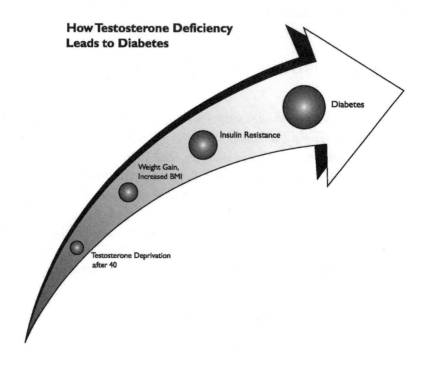

How Testosterone Deficiency Leads to Diabetes

Diabetes

Insulin Resistance

Weight Gain, Increased BMI

Testosterone Deprivation after 40

The terms associated with diabetes are confusing if you are not versed in medical terminology, so let's take a minute to define them.

Diabetes is a disease characterized by elevated blood sugar. In terms of diagnosing diabetes, doctors look at blood sugar levels over 100 when you are fasting, or 140 two hours after you have eaten. In contrast to the healthy, stable physiology of the body, elevated blood sugar causes progressive damage to your organs.

Type 1 diabetes is generally a disease of children and young adults that starts with a virus that affects the pancreas and destroys the hormone-producing cells that make insulin. These patients require insulin supplementation to survive.

Type 2 diabetes is a disease related to weight gain, obesity, hormone loss, age, and inactivity. It begins with insulin resistance, then evolves to conditions of low blood sugar, and finally results in inadequate insulin production.

Insulin resistance (or insensitivity) occurs when individual cells fail or resist absorption of sugar and insulin, which leads to an overproduction of insulin by the pancreas. Insulin from the pancreas delivers blood sugar into the cells so the sugar can be transformed into energy. With insulin resistance, the cell wall will not unlock the cell so the sugar can enter and be used as "food." As we get older or fatter, this process deteriorates, and our cells become insulin insensitive or immune, so the blood sugar that does not get into the cells "bounces off" and deposits as fat. It becomes easier to gain weight as we age because of insulin insensitivity.

Obesity is defined as a BMI (body mass index) greater than 30. The BMI formula is calculated by taking your weight (in pounds) and dividing it by your height in inches, squared. Then multiply that number by 703. Following is the formula: (weight in pounds ÷ [height in inches x height in inches]) x 703.

Hypoglycemia is caused by lowered levels of glucose in the blood, or blood sugar. Within 30 minutes to several hours after eating, your blood sugar levels drop below 65. This results in symptoms of drowsiness, dizziness, hunger, cravings for carbohydrates, and sometimes sweating.

Carbohydrates, or "carbs," are a type of food that breaks down into glucose in the stomach. Common examples are bread, pasta, cane sugar, brown sugar, rice, corn, oats, rye, fruits, and potatoes.

Normal Blood Sugar and Insulin Versus Type 2 Diabetes

The first step in becoming a type 2 diabetic is overreaction by the pancreas, which causes hypoglycemia (low blood sugar.) This causes a rapid cycling of insulin overproduction, which quickly drops blood sugar and is evidenced by hunger, fatigue, and headaches. This roller coaster of eating followed by low blood sugar creates a feast-and-famine process that denies the body the ability to maintain a stable energy source. These "harmonics" lead to both deprivation and excess. The excess blood sugar is stored as fat in the body, accelerating the process even further. It is, in other words, a vicious cycle. We spin further and further from stability and gain more and more weight. We are considered diabetic when our pancreas fails to produce insulin and blood sugar soars.

This process must be stopped to reverse the disease and requires weight loss and restriction of carbohydrates in the diet.

The Right Amount of Carbohydrates

The basis of popular diets like Atkins and South Beach is reducing carbohydrate intake. The maximum amount of carbs that can be eaten at one sitting without overstimulating insulin release is 25 grams. If someone eats 25 or fewer grams of carbs to control obesity, they should be able to lose weight until they achieve their ideal weight.

Learn to look at everything you eat or drink to determine the amount of carbs you're taking in. Be sure to look at both the total carbs and the fiber carbs. You can subtract the fiber amount from the total carbs because fiber passes directly through your body. The remainder turns to fat.

Essentially, the amount of carbs you eat controls blood sugar and insulin. The pancreas does the lion's share of the work by secreting insulin into the bloodstream during and after a meal, perfectly balancing the amount of food and carbohydrate in one feeding. If you eat more calories than your body requires, blood sugar is stored in the liver as glycogen or in the fatty tissues of the body.

Normal blood sugar management is meant to sustain you between meals. So ideally, you should eat a moderate amount of food, secrete just the right amount of insulin to use the energy in your food, and slowly pass the food into your intestines, which will increase the insulin slowly, deliver glucose to your tissues, and gradually drop the insulin and glucose back to normal before another meal. Basically, when you overeat and binge on carbs and other sugary foods, you're consuming too many carbohydrates and making too much insulin too quickly for your body to handle. The goal is to slow down the process of emptying the stomach so that you receive the right amount of insulin at a time. If you release insulin quickly, your blood sugar goes up quickly and then down to a very low level, which makes you feel tired, crabby, and hungry. This yo-yoing blood sugar leaves you completely drained at the end of the day, with an increase in body fat to boot!

As we noted earlier, our cells must be "sensitive" to insulin in order to accept and absorb blood sugar to make energy. Our blood sugar travels into the cells "piggy-backed" on insulin; otherwise it cannot be received and used. Insulin insensitivity blocks the admission of glucose into the cell, and no energy can be made. Worse yet, the blood sugar that is rejected is sent to the fat to be stored.

Unless you are very active on a daily basis, eat properly, maintain an ideal body weight, and replace missing hormones, this system tends to break down in midlife. If you are not active, you gain fat, causing your cells to become insensitive, and you become prediabetic.

If you think glucose control in your body is complicated, the malfunction of that system is even more so. It is a complex process, but it all occurs without your conscious assistance. There are, however, a few things you can consciously do to avoid diabetes:

- Avoid damage to the pancreas.
- Avoid heavy alcohol use.
- Avoid overeating carbohydrates, especially grains, rice, and sugar.
- Exercise!
- Get tested for gallstones.
- Get treated with testosterone replacement if you have a deficiency.
- Treat insulin sensitivity with the drug metformin.
- Treat menopause with nonoral estradiol replacement.

Avoiding the habits and getting treated for the conditions that lead to diabetes will require effort on your part. Careful meal planning, ample exercise, and monitoring of metabolism, testosterone, and weight are all necessary. Once blood sugar has increased beyond normal and the symptoms of prediabetes occur (hypoglycemic episodes), reversing the progressive condition of diabetes is much like throwing a rope to someone who is sliding down the face of a steep cliff and pulling them back up and away from the edge. It can be done, but it's not easy!

The First Step in Developing Type 2 Diabetes

Insulin resistance is the precursor to type 2 diabetes and is often called hypoglycemia. It is a genetic and hormone-regulated imbalance characterized by the inefficient use of glucose (blood sugar) for energy because of insensitivity to insulin. The condition makes it impossible to use the food you eat to make energy. Insulin resistance runs in families and especially in women who have polycystic ovarian disease, but it can be treated to prevent diabetes.

The symptoms of insulin resistance also include swelling, persistent weight gain that is unresponsive to dieting, and an increase in abdominal fat. The old carbohydrate-rich food pyramid that the USDA once recommended for us has made insulin resistance an epidemic today. The more simple carbohydrates we eat, the worse it gets as we gain weight from those valueless foods. Luckily, there is now a new food pyramid (technically a food plate) introduced by nutrition experts at Harvard, and it's gaining momentum among dietitians and nutritionists. The Healthy Eating Plate consists of half fruits and veggies, one-quarter protein, and the remaining quarter whole grains.

How to Find Out If You Have Insulin Resistance

You may suspect that you have insulin resistance if you have episodes of fatigue and weakness several hours after a meal. It can be determined through blood sugar and insulin tests taken before and after a glucose-rich meal.

Blood test results in the following values will indicate insulin resistance and diabetes. Testing for insulin resistance requires:

☐ Fasting blood insulin and glucose testing

- High blood insulin: >10
- Low blood sugar: <60
- Hb (hemoglobin) A1c: <5.7% (normal)

☐ Fasting lipids = high triglycerides: >150 mg/dl
☐ Inflammation (C-reactive protein) = elevated: >3.0

Medically, insulin resistance is diagnosed by researching family and medical history, testing, and trial of an insulin-resistance medication in combination with a meal plan of six small meals per day with very low carbohydrates. If left untreated, insulin resistance will progress to type 2 diabetes, heart disease, obesity, severe fatigue, and chronic infections. Trust me—you don't want these problems! It is much better to prevent them because there is no real turning back once you have full-blown type 2 diabetes (unless you are a candidate for bariatric surgery).

Treatment Options for Insulin Resistance

If you already have prediabetes or diabetes, there are medications that can help you. Among these are metformin and rosiglitazone. Rosiglitazone and Actos are only currently approved for diabetes, but they work fairly well for insulin resistance and prevention of diabetes. (This is another legal off-label use of an FDA-approved drug.) Actos is also optional, but does not produce good weight reduction. The newest drug approved for diabetes is the daily shot Victoza. It is not insulin but works on the liver to slow release of glycogen, slows the rate of passage of food from the stomach to the intestines, decreases insulin resistance, and suppresses hunger. It is currently being evaluated for approval by the FDA for prediabetes and weight loss.

As we've said, imbalanced hormones, a sedentary lifestyle, poor diet, and obesity all lead to insulin resistance. The standard medical therapy is metformin (in the long-acting form), which makes cells porous to glucose and insulin, letting them in to make energy instead of fat. Balancing hormones, using metformin or Victoza, weight loss, and a healthier lifestyle can prevent the progression to overt diabetes.

Diabetes is not just another condition. It is an all-consuming disease that accelerates aging and robs you of your quality of life by damaging blood vessels, causing heart disease, and increasing weight gain and blood pressure. And it puts you at risk for many other diseases. It is well worth the work to pull yourself up the cliff toward normal weight and blood sugar control. It will save you time in the long run. You do not want to be tethered to an insulin pen or a refrigerator for an insulin supply for the remainder of your life.

HEART DISEASE AND STROKE

We always concentrate on our risks for breast cancer, yet annually more women die of vascular disease and stroke. We need to protect ourselves as best we can from developing diseases of the heart and blood vessels.

In medicine, we often encounter a "serendipitous" effect in which we find the cure for one disease while looking for the cure for another. When Kathy began to treat women with bio-identical testosterone and estradiol pellets, stroke or heart disease weren't even on her radar. She just wanted to revitalize their lives in terms of cognition, weight loss issues, sex drive, and overall quality of life. She discovered that, while these issues were improved, the number of patients suffering from or showing risk factors for developing stroke and heart disease also diminished.

This is great news for all of us! The replacement of testosterone and estradiol can protect us from the basic malfunction that damages our vessels as we age: the development of plaque, or "corrosion," on our blood vessels that decreases blood flow and causes disease. The simple formula for making plaque (also known as arteriosclerosis) is as follows:

$$\text{LDL cholesterol} + \text{triglycerides} + \text{inflammation} = \text{vascular damage} = \text{plaque}$$

Estradiol and testosterone work to decrease total and LDL cholesterol ("bad cholesterol") and increase HDL cholesterol ("good cholesterol"). They also decrease inflammation in the vessels, working to keep your "pipes clean" and prevent vascular diseases that lead to problems like heart attack and stroke.

The Imbalance That Causes Heart Disease and Stroke

Heart disease is not really a disease of the heart muscle itself, but rather a disease of the arteries, blood vessels that supply the heart with blood. These vital pipelines supply the constantly beating heart with oxygen and glucose. Progressive buildup of cholesterol plaque over many years gets thicker and thicker until it narrows the arteries, so much so that the heart is stressed when we exercise. (One of the signs of vascular heart disease is shortness of breath.) When our heart becomes impaired by narrowing arteries, the rest of our body is impaired, too. However, the heart is much more important to our survival, so it is discussed more frequently.

The next vital area of concern is the carotid arteries in the neck that supply the brain with its necessary oxygen and nutrients. When they are compromised we may experience a stroke, memory loss, or both.

The last two areas of importance when we have narrowed arteries are the aorta and the iliac vessels leading to the lower legs and feet. The aorta collects plaque and narrows the vessels to the kidneys, leading to decreased kidney function. The aorta also leads to the iliac arteries, which supply the pelvis and legs. Poor color or healing in the lower legs, as well as pain with exercise or at rest in the legs, is called claudication and results from poor blood flow.

This comparison of cross-sections of healthy and atherosclerotic arteries shows the thickened vessel walls and the narrowed diameter of the artery after years' worth of cholesterol plaque has built up on the vessel walls.

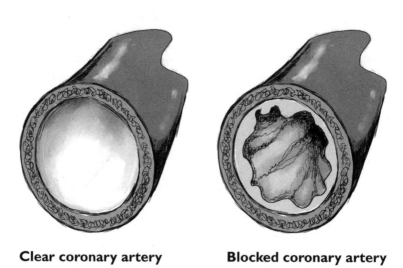

Clear coronary artery   **Blocked coronary artery**

It is bad enough that vessels are damaged by cholesterol plaques and impair the flow of blood, but these same vessels lose their elasticity and can no longer dilate when we need more blood flow to an area. This leads to elevated blood pressure.

The Role of Cholesterol

It would seem that cholesterol is the bad guy in all of this, but it is also a necessary building block for our cells, our brain, and all of our steroid hormones (estradiol, testosterone, progesterone, cortisol, aldosterone, and others). When cholesterol works in an environment of hormone balance, it is an asset to our body. Cholesterol plays the role of villain after TDS and menopause; when our bodies become inflamed from lack of testosterone, we gain weight and become inactive. Under these circumstances, cholesterol begins to stick to the walls of our arteries, causing vascular disease and eventually heart disease or stroke.

Total and LDL cholesterol and triglyceride elevation alone do not cause disease because these cholesterols slide right by the vessel walls and do not stick. It is inflammation that instigates the cholesterol deposition on vessels by making the vessels "sticky" to cholesterol. Thus, neither elevated cholesterol nor inflammation alone harm vessels and lead to the disease; both are required.

Vascular Disease: Symptoms and Risk Factors

In women, vascular disease is marked by:

- Damage to the blood vessels
- Decreased HDL cholesterol
- Elevated LDL cholesterol
- Elevated triglycerides
- Inflammation
- Lack of nitric oxide
- Lack of oxygenation to the tissues

Diet, exercise, omega-3 acids, niacin, selenium, folic acid, and CoQ 10 as well as testosterone and estradiol can prevent or rectify these problems. Hormone deficiency can increase your risk, but other genetic and lifestyle factors can also come into play, including family history of heart disease, menopause and TDS, smoking, inactivity, obesity, alcohol use, junk food, diabetes, insulin resistance, and hypertension.

These risk factors—excluding smoking, inactivity, and poor diet—are common with menopause and TDS. Hormone loss is pivotal in all of the other risk factors and is relatively easy to treat. Therefore it is very critical in your quest for health that you receive hormone replacement if needed.

Tests That Indicate You Are at Risk

After menopause, women should be evaluated for vascular disease through several tests, including blood tests, blood pressure, stress echocardiogram, possibly a "pure scan" CT to detect calcification of the vessels of the heart, examining the carotid arteries, and a cardiology exam, all on a regular and ongoing basis. Blood tests include:

- 8 A.M. cortisol
- Cardiac CRP—tests for inflammation
- CBC
- Fasting blood sugar and HbA1c
- Fasting insulin
- Free testosterone and estradiol and FSH (follicle-stimulating hormone) levels
- Homocysteine
- Lipids—for cholesterol (HDL and LDL) and triglycerides

These blood tests will reveal your risk for heart disease and stroke and allow your doctor to follow your risk factors yearly and treat you accordingly.

Finding a Preventive Solution

Unfortunately, we currently have several roadblocks to a successful prevention program for heart disease and stroke. Medicine has only recently recognized the substantial gender differences in the symptoms of heart disease in women; most ER doctors still look for the male symptoms of a heart attack, which leaves women who have the disease underdiagnosed. Unlike men, women experience back pain, jaw pain, nausea, bloating, numbness, and fatigue—in addition to the gender-neutral symptoms of pain down the left arm, chest pressure, sweating, and shortness of breath. Men usually complain of pain radiating down their left arm and that they feel like they have an elephant standing on their chest.

Medicine is only starting to understand the gender difference in risk factors that contribute to vascular disease and heart damage. Men have always been considered to be at risk for heart disease, so medicine pays close attention to their risk factors. Women generally do not start developing vascular damage until after they turn 40 when testosterone loss, weight gain, and insulin resistance begin, and the vascular accumulation of plaque accelerates at menopause. Doctors miss the beginning of the problem because the current thought only considers women at risk when we pass through menopause. By then women are already on their way to nonreversible plaque in their blood vessels, so it's too late to take preventive, life-saving action.

It is no use to worry about these problems unless you know how to prevent them. There are three categories of preventive measures a woman can take to improve her odds:

1. Nutritional supplementation
2. Medication
3. Lifestyle changes

Let's take a look at these categories individually.

Nutritional supplementation that decreases cholesterol and inflammation is available over the counter. If you have a family history of vascular diseases, we encourage you to take these countermeasures.

- To decrease cholesterol levels:
    - CoQ 10
    - Fish oil
    - Vitamin A and D
    - Vitamin C

- To decrease inflammation:
    - A nutritional supplement like Vemma
    - A resveratrol supplement
    - Fish oil
    - Flaxseed oil
    - Vitamin D

Medications your doctor may suggest to improve your cholesterol and inflammatory state include:

- 81 mg aspirin
- Antihypertensives
- Beta blockers
- Celebrex
- Diuretics
- Estradiol pellets or other bio-identical estradiol in nonoral form
- Metformin
- Statins
- Replacement hormones (estradiol and testosterone)
- Testosterone pellets or other bio-identical testosterone in nonoral form
- Thyroid hormone replacement
- Victoza

Lifestyle changes may include:

- A low-carb diet to decrease weight and insulin resistance
- A wheat-free (gluten-free) diet to decrease inflammation
- De-stressing with meditation, yoga, or relaxation tapes
- Exercise: 20 minutes daily or one hour three times a week
- Limiting yourself to one alcoholic drink per day
- Quitting smoking or use of drugs (such as cocaine or methamphetamine)

If in addition to discussing medications with your doctor, you can change your lifestyle and add supplements, you are on your way to preventing these killers of a quality life!

Remember that there are other cardiac problems such as an arrhythmia, infection, or malfunction of the heart muscle that impair heart function but are unrelated to the heart's vascular system. For other heart concerns, you need to see a cardiologist for diagnosis and treatment. Our primary goals are to change your thinking about your risk of heart disease and stroke, and provide vital information you can use when speaking with a physician.

Evidence for the Effectiveness of Estrogen and Testosterone Replacement

While hormone replacement has been studied in the past, and in many cases study results supported the efficacy of testosterone and estrogen, these findings were rarely publicized outside the medical community. The evidence for the use of hormone therapy in women who are at risk for heart disease is strong and makes physiologic sense: hormones are antioxidants that repair damaged vascular cells, preventing vascular disease.

When treating women with testosterone and estradiol pellets, we see a difference in as little as three months. This is because these two hormones utilize their antioxidant properties to cause the body to use cholesterol for growth and hormone production instead of allowing it to circulate at high levels and deposit on blood vessels. Estradiol also dilates blood vessels, decreasing blood pressure. Estrogen also improves the secretion of extra salt from the kidneys, which lowers blood pressure and reduces the stress that high blood pressure puts on the heart.

The revised results of the Women's Health Initiative (WHI) study published in 2010 conceded that estrogen alone improves cholesterol levels and decreases the incidence of vascular disease in aging women. The original study was confusing and implicated estradiol in the cause of heart disease. The new study corrects these results and shows estradiol is the "good guy."

The importance of testosterone in the prevention of obesity was described in a review of the literature by Odette Evangelista and Mary Ann McLaughlin, published in the *Review of Cardiovascular Risk Factors in Women, Gender Medicine 2009*. This review revealed that testosterone replacement resulted in more lean body mass, less abdominal obesity, and lower inflammation, all of which translated into lower risk for vascular disease.

The important thing to remember is this: heart disease and stroke do not happen only to other people. They are likely to happen to you unless you take precautions to prevent them. You can reduce your risk and increase your future quality of life if you follow our suggestions, change your habits, and balance your hormones. You have the power!

Now that we have examined both the immediate symptoms and the long-term illnesses that are impacted by the loss of testosterone, let's look at the next two hormones to go in the aging cascade. As we move into an examination of progesterone and estrogen, we want to emphasize that it would not be advisable to consider only replacing progesterone or estrogen without considering testosterone replacement as well. Testosterone lowers cholesterol and decreases inflammation, and as you've seen, it is the initial or foundational hormone to replace to prevent the cascade of illnesses in the aging process.

Your hormones work in tandem to keep your system in balance. As you will learn in the next chapter, progesterone has a major role in the lives of women who are not menopausal. It is important as a balancing hormone because of the extreme swings that estrogen can make when a woman is cycling. Once a woman has gone through menopause, progesterone becomes important only as a tool for controlling bleeding from the uterus. It is no longer a whole body–balancing hormone. If a woman has a hysterectomy or uses a Mirena IUD, she does not need progesterone after menopause. The last hormone we will discuss after progesterone is estrogen. It is a whole-body hormone secondary in importance to testosterone in women's mental, physical, and emotional health.

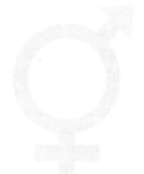

CHAPTER 7

Progesterone Deficiency and Estradiol Loss

In this book, we have spent much time explaining why testosterone replacement is the critical first step in the replacement of hormones in order to prevent the diseases of aging. Now it's time to look at the other two female hormones that are involved in the aging process: progesterone and estrogen.

Generally, we recommend that most women replace their testosterone when it is lost, and replace their estradiol. If a woman has a uterus, it may also be necessary for her to replace her progesterone. Let's start by talking about why that is.

The Second Step of Aging: Progesterone Loss

Progesterone is the hormone that predominates when we are pregnant. It is unique to women, it is necessary to prevent estrogen dominance because it balances estradiol, and it prevents PMS. It decreases with age after 40 and usually after testosterone drops to a critical level. Progesterone deficiency is called many things, but the most common problem associated with progesterone loss is PMS.

Progesterone deficiency is characterized by an inability to fall asleep, irritability and anxiety, depression, and breast tenderness and swelling. Some patients exhibited irregular uterine bleeding, multiple miscarriages, retention of fluid, and bloating and slowing of the GI tract. Progesterone deficiency also offsets or balances the symptoms of estrogen dominance and decreases cravings.

There is a cultural myth that PMS is natural to women because they are viewed as more "emotional," "reactive," and "unstable" than men. The myth has it that every 28 days or so women go crazy. This is supposed to be beyond their control, so everyone in their sphere of influence can only duck and cover until the storm has passed. If *men* had this reputation, medicine probably would have found a solution to PMS long ago!

For many years, PMS was considered merely a psychiatric problem, unrelated to hormones. It wasn't until the 1990s that alternative doctors initially suspected that a hormonal imbalance— specifically a lack of progesterone—caused this condition. Being willing to challenge the status quo and test new treatments, Kathy began treating women who had PMS with pure bio-identical progesterone and vitamins containing large amounts of magnesium— with great results. Yet despite her high success rate, mainstream medicine dismissed this treatment as crazy.

A compounding pharmacist named Pete Hueseman, RPh, PD, helped Kathy develop the treatment. In the beginning, she prescribed progesterone in the form of rectal suppositories, then vaginal suppositories, progressing to vaginal tabs. She currently prefers sublingual (under the tongue) tablets or pure progesterone pellets that are placed below the skin. These two methods avoid what is known as the "first-pass effect": the metabolic breakdown that happens when medicines are absorbed first in the stomach and then processed through the liver. When this happens, the concentration of the drug is greatly decreased.

Today, the loss of progesterone is a widely researched and confirmed source of PMS. Despite these definitive findings, the American Congress of Obstetricians and Gynecologists still does not consider PMS to be a condition related to the loss of progesterone. Hence, it does not recognize the addition of natural progesterone between days 14 and 28 as an effective treatment. If an OB/GYN applicant for fellowship cites progesterone insufficiency as the cause of PMS on the national board exam and indicates natural progesterone as the treatment, that answer will be marked incorrect. Yet Kathy's 20-plus years of practice in the field, many research studies, and the work of other practicing OB/GYNs have demonstrated the cause of PMS and the efficacy of progesterone supplementation by treating millions of women with PMS. They are not crazy, just "progesterone-ally" impaired!

ASK BRETT

"All my life I've heard people make jokes about PMS and women. Anytime I am moody, upset, or depressed, my husband dismisses me by saying I am having PMS! I just hate it. Women are always challenged and belittled this way. I want to know from your perspective: are women more emotionally volatile and unstable? Are we raving emotional bio-hazards because of PMS?" —Kim, 32

Kim, all of us, both men and women, are raving emotional biohazards when our hormones are out of balance. I know many men who have been flooded with rage and acted out in ways that were harmful to the people they loved or society in general. What do you think happens when someone experiences road rage? It is the same stuff. There is no technical exclusion of men from this process. Women have just gotten a bum rap over the years. It's common knowledge that during the time leading up to a woman's period, her hormones are in flux, and society uses that as an excuse to blame and dismiss your concerns. You don't have to put up with it. You can also look into treatments to reduce the intensity of those mood fluctuations.

PROGESTERONE: BUT WHAT DOES IT DO, EXACTLY?

Like other female hormones, progesterone has many roles to play in a woman's life and health. Women start producing progesterone when they begin to cycle and ovulate. The ovary only produces progesterone during the second half of the menstrual cycle (days 14 to 28) and during pregnancy. It is not produced prior to the beginning of menstruation or after menopause, and it is not generally needed then either. It is similar to time-released medicine, beginning and stopping at certain developmental points. The only exception to this is when a woman is pregnant, because during pregnancy, progesterone is the dominant hormone in the female system. At all other times, progesterone production and delivery follow the cycle of ovulation.

Like estradiol and testosterone, progesterone is produced in the ovary, or more specifically, in the tissue from which the egg has ovulated (the corpus luteum). This is why it is only secreted after ovulation each month on day 14 and until day 28, when this tissue wears out. When progesterone drops precipitously before a period, it instigates bleeding from the lining of the uterus.

Normal Progesterone Levels Before Age 40
Day 21 = 10–25 nanograms/milliliter

Progesterone is also the one female hormone that calms women emotionally, reducing anxiety and depression and lessening mood swings. It is their "mellow out" hormone. For example, progesterone bestows a calming feeling during pregnancy when the normal flow of estrogen and testosterone, which help women focus and have energy for running their lives, is redirected to the development and maintenance of the life of the fetus. The manufacturing of progesterone that is not devoted to preserving the pregnancy shifts to the placenta, but the happy side effect of this process is that the woman feels calmer.

Progesterone Imbalances

Stress, starvation, trauma, illness, social problems—all these can negatively impact the ability of a woman to become pregnant or carry a baby to term. Progesterone is a tool of nature that allows us to become pregnant or stay pregnant past the first trimester when we are under severe stress. When women are not in a position to have children, they stop producing enough progesterone. In the world of "survival of the species," fertility is one of the first systems to shut down, saving resources for human beings who are already living.

Modern women in civilized cultures face stressors that impact their biological responses to the environment in ways that are similar to their more primitive sisters' experiences. Much of this stress, which is significant and constant for many young women, is socially generated. Women today deal with issues of relational bullying among other women; anxiety about self-image and body image; the challenges of finding a home, meeting a husband, and having children of their own; and planning a future during times that are inherently difficult. This all causes us to sometimes experience the same adaptive adjustments as women in a primitive tribe: their progesterone levels often fluctuate, or even cease, as a result of the accumulated stressors of modern life.

Replacing Progesterone Is to PMS as Replacing Insulin Is to Diabetes

One of the discussions physicians often have with their patients involves using medicines to treat or correct chemical or hormonal imbalances. A cultural myth in the United States maintains that taking medicines for mood-related issues is a character flaw. It's not.

Physicians who understand the true nature of PMS and mood disorders often offer diabetes as an analogy to their patients. "Would you encourage a diabetic needing insulin to take it and get better," they ask, "or just tough it out because being tough shows character?"

The patient invariably says, "Take the insulin."

"So," the doctor's reasoning continues, "what if mood disorders were chemical, hormonal, or disease based rather than a function of weak character? Should we restore the missing ingredient, or should you just tough it out?"

We see no merit in the traditional philosophy of "just tough it out." There is both scientific and anecdotal evidence to build the case that women who suffer from shortages of their natural hormones, in particular testosterone and progesterone, need to have them replaced. This replacement benefits their health and protects them from multiple ill effects of aging. Why should we ignore the problem just because the treatment is not something that has always been done?

Does Everyone Need Progesterone?

Every day in the office we hear, "Do I need progesterone replacement *after menopause*?" This is really several questions lumped together for which there is no blanket answer that applies to all women.

Let's simplify the answer so you can apply it to your own situation. Progesterone, which all women make prior to their 40s, is designed to prepare the uterus for the implantation of an egg after fertilization and in preparation for pregnancy. That is the primary purpose of progesterone as a hormone when you're young.

A secondary biological purpose for progesterone is to protect the uterus from overstimulation by estradiol. If estradiol is left unchecked or unbalanced by progesterone, the uterine lining will become so thick that it vastly increases the likelihood of uterine cancers. Progesterone, therefore, keeps the uterine lining stable by preventing estrogen from increasing the lining's thickness, which leads to abnormality.

Because progesterone naturally protects a single organ, the uterus, doctors replace progesterone in every woman who possesses a uterus (has not had a hysterectomy) or who has not had an ablation (a procedure that burns out the lining of the uterus) with an oral synthetic progesteronelike chemical called a progestin. Unfortunately, these oral pills do *not* have the same effect on the uterus or PMS as natural, nonoral progesterone. Oral progestins are transformed in the liver into several chemicals, the most risky of which is estrone, which we refer to as "old lady" estrogen. This is a hormone to avoid, as it makes women feel and look old.

Because synthetic progestins are so dissimilar from natural progesterone, the only safe choice is bio-identical nonoral progesterone.

After menopause we do not require progesterone to balance estradiol replacement for two reasons. First, replacement of estradiol is generally given in the same dose every day. Progesterone is needed to balance the variable level of estradiol produced during the menstrual cycle. Second, the dosage of estradiol is very much lower after menopause; therefore, the blood level is lower.

When women hit menopause, they can control the amount of estradiol that is circulating in the bloodstream. Balancing estradiol with progesterone is much easier in menopausal women than premenopausal women, who make a different amount of estradiol daily. For women in menopause, PMS is no longer an issue, so there is no hormonal reason to support the use of progesterone in menopausal women without a uterus. So, as I mentioned earlier, the reason we give progesterone to menopausal women is to keep their uterus safe from too much buildup of lining, which may become cancerous over a long period of time.

The one exception to this rule is for a small percentage of women who need progesterone to calm them and balance their neurotransmitters. Unlike most women, who can replace their testosterone and estradiol to premenopausal levels without getting PMS, some women still continue to suffer from irritability and insomnia and require progesterone even without a uterus and after menopause. We diagnose these women by exclusion, evaluating their symptoms as they respond to testosterone and estradiol treatment, in order to balance their hormone dosage. If they still experience depression, irritability, and trouble falling asleep after adequate hormone doses, we add a low dose of natural nonoral progesterone. The result is a resolution of all of their menopause and TDS symptoms, as well as those from PMS. After they receive all three hormones, their neurotransmitters are stabilized and they receive the full effects of testosterone and estradiol replacement.

Why Progesterone Works Better Than Antidepressants for PMS

Patients express so much relief when they are told that there is a natural and an effective treatment for PMS. They are so happy to hear that being an "emotional wreck" stems from a simple hormonal imbalance, one that is also treatable.

As we said earlier, PMS has been ignored for years by the medical community and considered a psychiatric issue. Therefore, it is usually treated with antidepressants that fight its *symptoms* instead of treating its hormone-based *cause*. This approach is laughably ineffective. It's almost tragic, really, when there are a variety of very effective treatments available using bio-identical progesterone and/or testosterone.

The three options for bio-identical hormone treatment of PMS include:

- Bio-identical testosterone treatment given as a pellet every four months, or as a vaginal tablet nightly, as it relieves many of the symptoms of PMS

- Natural sublingual (held under the tongue), buccal (held in the cheek), or vaginal transdermal progesterone during days 14 to 28 of the menstrual cycle

- Progesterone pellets given once every four months to create a constant low level of progesterone to balance estradiol levels

All effective treatments with these two bio-identical hormones are nonoral because taking progesterone or testosterone in any form orally, even bio-identical hormones, breaks it down into estrogens, complicates the problem, and worsens the symptoms. In Chapter 9, we'll go into more detail on these various treatment options.

Progesterone Treatment Recommendations

There are a few treatment parameters that make progesterone replacement more effective and decrease the risks of side effects:

- You should only take bio-identical progesterone. Everything else is a progestin, an artificial synthetic that makes things worse, as the Women's Health Initiative study of 2002 demonstrated.

- When treating PMS, you should take nonoral forms of bio-identical progesterone (compounded), because oral forms go through the first-pass effect and are metabolized differently by the digestive system, creating harmful by-products.

- Administer bio-identical progesterone at night, in a 24-hour dosage, because it will make you sleepy.

- Avoid multiple dosing throughout the day because progesterone induces fatigue, low blood sugar, and unpredictable blood levels.

Recommended Dosages

- Subdermal pellets administered every 4 months
- Transdermal creams, 4 to 6 times a day
- Vaginal and sublingual tablets, generally once a day
- Vaginal or rectal suppositories, generally twice a day

To treat PMS, administration can be daily throughout the month or only on days 14 to 28 of the menstrual cycle. For menopausal women progesterone is not cycled.

Having learned about testosterone and progesterone, next we'll look at the third hormone in the aging cascade, estrogen. Estrogen is particularly interesting because of all the myths around menopause. We will take a close look at the three types of estrogen: estrone, estradiol, and estriol.

You may have questions about the symptoms that define menopause. We will answer those and focus on the different treatment options for replacing estrogen. What are the risks and benefits of the different methods of estrogen replacement? What if you have blood clotting issues? Is it always necessary to replace both estrogen and progesterone? These are common questions women ask every day. We want you and your doctor to have the latest information and thinking from the cutting edge of antiaging medicine.

THE THIRD STEP OF AGING: MENOPAUSE = ESTRADIOL LOSS

Menopause is the last step in aging, and it occurs when estradiol, the estrogen of youth, is no longer produced in the ovaries. It seems fitting that we should end our discussion of the aging cascade with its final stage, menopause.

It is important to discuss this particular hormone because there is so much controversy over estrogen replacement: if, when, and how it should be replaced. To make this subject more challenging, the published research often shows conflicting and confusing results. Patients naturally become reluctant to do anything to remedy their menopausal symptoms—for fear of doing the wrong thing.

In this section, we provide the most *current* research so you can make an educated decision for yourself with an understanding of the myths, misconceptions, and various options for estrogen replacement therapy.

The Ins and Outs of Estrogen

Estradiol is the primary estrogen that makes us look and feel young and feminine. But it is not quite that simple, because women make a total of *three* estrogens over a lifetime and each has a different role and chemical activity.

1. **Estradiol** (E2) from the ovary: provides the "female" figure, waistline, soft skin, perky breasts, wet vagina, elasticity of the skin and vagina, thick and shiny head hair, low lipid profile, clear thinking, and elevated mood

2. **Estriol** (E3) from the placenta: pregnancy estrogen, weakly estrogenic, helps skin and hair grow, increases the deposit of fat for storage for breast feeding, and is a marker of placental health

3. **Estrone** (E1) from the adrenal gland: "old lady" estrogen, contributes to belly fat, sagging and painful breasts, breast cancer, loss of memory, fatigue, diminished mood, irritability, obesity, and sagging skin

Just for clarity's sake, when we refer to menopause and loss of "estrogen" in the rest of the book, we are only referring to *estradiol*.

Menopause: Fact and Fiction

Conventional wisdom is a term used to reflect what people generally think or feel about a topic. It is not necessarily right or wrong; it is not based on facts—it's just what people seem to "know" and "say." Menopause is often subject to conventional wisdom.

The Internet, the news media, and information that spreads without anyone really knowing its source or accuracy all add to our confusion and misunderstanding about the realities of menopause. Because of this complexity, many women rely on word of mouth among their girlfriends to come up with a course of action. This is not likely to lead to a best outcome. So much information in the zone of conventional wisdom about menopause is simply wrong, yet often repeated. Social scientists refer to this as "the big lie": when something is said often enough and loudly enough, eventually people come to believe it, even when it is not true.

Our confusion about menopause often stems from medical studies conducted by drug companies or federal agencies for the purpose of reaching a particular result, and who profit if misinformation is believed. Or they are conducted by people who are motivated to act in a certain way. People are persuaded to take or not take a drug based on a contrived result.

When Kathy was in medical school, she once heard a joke about medical research:

"When you do research for a pharmaceutical company, what is the most important question to ask the chief investigator or investor in that research?"

"What do you want the results of the study to conclude?"

Sadly, it is true that data can be used to say what someone wants it to say. All it takes is manipulating how the study is done or the variables of the study. Most people are not trained to tell good research from bad. When a study concludes a particular "truth," before we believe it, we have learned to ask, "Who did the research and why? Who is making the money?"

There is a lot of information on menopause out there, and some of it is valuable. But it's a challenge to find it, evaluate it, and plan a course of action based on what is scientific and verifiable.

As a policy, Kathy compares research outcomes with the clinical findings of her 25 years in OB/GYN practice. That is how she knew immediately that the WHI study (the notorious 2002 study that scared doctors and their patients into thinking that estrogen replacement caused breast cancer and heart disease) was wrong; in her practice there were as many patients who took estrogen and got breast cancer as there were who *never* took estrogen replacement and got breast cancer. There was no statistical difference! Current studies now discount the initial WHI study and agree with Kathy's review of it.

Let's put an end to the madness of misinformation about estrogen replacement and place some facts before you, based on reliable research that has *no* vested interest in study outcomes.

The Facts about Estrogen Replacement

Let's start with the definition of menopause. Even that is confusing. Menopause can be interpreted as a "point in time" when you have not had a period for a year or have had your ovaries removed. It can be considered the phase of your life following that point in time that represents the end of your ability to become pregnant. Of course, a definition is not real life, and menopause does not occur in most women when they simply cease to have periods for a year. The ways in which menopause presents itself vary with the individual, and women experience the end of reproduction in different ways.

If you have joined the battalions of women who share the menopause experience, you certainly have heard more stories about menopause than you could have concocted in your imagination. A few of the scenarios that are most common include the advent of menopause after years of irregular cycles, or menses stopping abruptly with no warning. Menopause can occur while periods are still cycling, and a blood test reveals an elevated FSH, indicating the absence of eggs in the ovary. There are many roads that lead to the same place called menopause. Menopause can also occur when both ovaries are surgically removed, which is a very different path for entering menopause.

We diagnose menopause by ordering a blood test that measures FSH (a pituitary hormone). When this hormone is greater than 23 milliunits per liter, for two tests taken two weeks apart, then a woman is considered menopausal and infertile, and can stop birth control. Before menopause, the FSH level varies on a daily basis, and after menopause, it is generally stable day to day. When we replace estradiol after menopause, our goal is to supply enough estradiol to suppress FSH and achieve a level below 23 milliunits per liter, which is associated with resolution of the symptoms of menopause.

FSH Blood Levels
Follicle-Stimulating Hormone

- FSH blood levels vary during the menstrual cycle

- Test FSH during the first seven days after bleeding starts (days 1–7 of the menstrual cycle)

- Normal premenopause blood levels:
    - FSH = 3–23 MIU/ml

- Postmenopausal without estrogen replacement
    - Any day of month = >23 MIU/ml

The roads that lead to menopause are complicated. To set the record straight, the following statements are *factual:*

- Menopause begins one year after the last period.
- Menopause begins when the measurement of the FSH hormone is >23 MIU/ml twice over the course of two tests two weeks apart.
- Menopause also begins when a woman's ovaries are removed.
- Menopause begins the last stage of a woman's life.
- Many symptoms are attributed to menopause, but it is not defined by these symptoms. (Having hot flashes does not mean you are menopausal, even though they are one of the symptoms of menopause.)
- After menopause, you cannot become fertile again.

- The only estrogen that goes away at menopause is estradiol.

At this point we can hear you saying, "What about the things my mom told me about menopause?" In truth, most moms tell us what they know about menopause, but they may not have been accurately informed, either. Many of the misconceptions that follow are in the realm of old wives' tales because they have been passed down through generations to us, changing a little with each telling. Maybe you have heard these slices of misinformation from your female family members or from friends.

Current *misconceptions* about menopause include:

- Menopause starts and then stops, and your ovaries start working again.
- You can still get pregnant (with your own egg) after you have gone through menopause.
- Menopause stops when hot flashes stop.
- Hot flashes will spontaneously cease without treatment.
- After menopause, if a woman bleeds for any reason, on or off hormones, then she is out of menopause and is fertile again.
- Menopause just goes away.

We hope most of you are laughing, but Kathy has been asked questions based on these misconceptions throughout her career as a gynecologist. There are ways to cause bleeding, and you might transplant an embryo from a younger woman to allow a pregnancy, but menopause still remains the loss of ovarian fertility; no medical procedure can alter that.

The Symptoms of Menopause—Another Common Misconception

Common wisdom holds that menopause is all about hot flashes and dry vaginas and that sex drive is related to estrogen. Let's look at some real data about what the symptoms of menopause are and are not.

Symptoms of Estradiol Deficiency (Menopause)

- Hot flashes or flushes
- Dry vagina causing painful intercourse
- Fragile skin outside the vagina and throughout the body
- Thinning hair
- Osteoporosis
- Memory problems
- Sagging, dry skin
- Arthritis
- Interrupted sleep
- Urinary incontinence
- Vaginal infections

It's amazing how many of the symptoms of menopause are mixed up in these conversations with the symptoms of testosterone deprivation syndrome. The fact is that doctors and researchers lump the symptoms of estradiol loss (menopause) and testosterone loss (TDS) under the heading of "menopause" in statements to the press, and many such statements are based on outdated information. So how are women to understand the difference in their symptoms if their doctors don't? Surprisingly, many studies on "menopause" study the effectiveness of the replacement of estradiol for symptoms such as loss of libido, which is related to only testosterone.

For comparison, we are going to list the symptoms of menopause (loss of E2) and the symptoms of TDS (loss of testosterone) side by side.

Comparison of Symptoms

SYMPTOM	MENOPAUSE	TDS
Anxiety attacks	X	X
Decreased oil in skin		X
Decreased/loss of orgasms		X
Depression	X	X
Dry skin	X	X
Frequent urinary tract infections	X	
Frequent yeaset infections	X	
Hot flashes/night sweats	X	X
Hypoglycemia symptoms	X	
Increase in belly fat	X	X
Insomnia from hot flashes	X	
Irritable bladder	X	
Lack of menstrual periods for >1 year	X	
Loss of motivation		X
Loss of muscle mass	X	
Loss of sense of well-being	X	
Loss of sex drive		X
Loss of strength and stamina		X
Loss of vulvar and armpit hair		X
Memory loss	X	X
Mood problems	X	X
Osteoporosis	X	X
Shrinking clitoris		X
Stress urinary incontinence	X	
Uterine or vaginal prolapse	X	X
Vaginal dryness/painful intercourse	X	X
Weight gain	X	X

The two columns contain a few overlapping symptoms, but the symptoms on the left are typical in menopause and those on the right may occur much earlier when TDS occurs, sometime after the age of 40.

Symptoms Are Warning Signs: Know the Risks

Symptoms are warning signs that something is medically wrong, and they should not be ignored. They should always be investigated because, in most cases, the cause of the symptom is a harmful process that should be treated. When it comes to symptoms of menopause, however, mainstream medicine has told us to live with the symptoms and ignore their warnings.

Why is that?

Kathy believes that the medical community has ignored the diseases that these symptoms herald because they affect only women, because they are common, and because doctors do not know what to do about them. We should always investigate symptoms of diseases and then treat them to avoid subsequent illness.

Ignoring symptoms of menopause does not make it any less dangerous. Consider the hot flashes and night sweats that indicate the loss of estradiol. These symptoms are the result of a surge of the pituitary hormone FSH, which in turn causes a sympathetic (nervous system) surge, increasing heart rate and stimulating the stress centers, which in recent studies have been linked to an increased risk of heart attack. A heart attack is a severe medical problem that could be avoided by treating the hot flashes and night sweats at the outset with estradiol replacement!

Another common symptom of both TDS and menopause is weight gain, especially belly fat. This occurs at menopause because of the effect estradiol has on how we metabolize our calories. Many researchers have looked at this symptom and all have found that when estradiol deficiency occurs at menopause, it triggers the metabolic syndrome: weight gain, belly fat, insulin resistance, prediabetes, abnormal lipids with an increased level of triglycerides, and a decline of HDL cholesterol. Even if they are obese, women who are treated with estradiol for weight gain lose more belly fat than those who do not replace their estradiol. They are also less likely to develop prediabetes (insulin resistance). As we saw earlier in the book, diabetes and obesity are epidemic in the U.S., so wouldn't it be prudent to prevent the onset of diabetes in postmenopausal women through estrogen replacement?

Insomnia, another symptom of menopause, indicates more than just loss of estradiol and testosterone. Insomnia and the fatigue that follows result in mood changes, headaches, and loss of memory. Mood changes lead to depression and anxiety that require medication. Headaches are debilitating and require another host of medications.

Lastly, the loss of short-term recall caused by the loss of testosterone and estradiol indicates a loss of neurotransmitters that progresses to dementia, and sometimes Alzheimer's disease, as we touched on earlier. Since other diseases quickly follow the onset of menopause, preventing them by replacing estrogen makes much more sense than making a woman "tough it out" and end up with other conditions and diseases that require multiple drugs.

Every symptom of menopause is a warning sign for a disease or a dangerous condition that will inevitably occur unless estradiol, the hormone that is deficient, is replaced. If we treated hot flashes for women like we do chest pain for men, we would seek appropriate treatment.

Long-Term Benefits of Replacing Estradiol

The Journal of Clinical Endocrinology & Metabolism produced a very complete treatise on postmenopausal hormone therapy in July 2010. The findings were based on scientific research done in many specialties and vary according to the type of hormone replaced and the delivery system used. No matter how you interpret this compilation of research, estradiol offers great advantages as a preventive treatment for many debilitating diseases of aging.

HRT (hormone replacement therapy) means **estrogen of any type, plus progestin** combined in a postmenopausal medication for women. (HRT can also refer to testosterone, but this is the common usage.)

ERT (estrogen replacement therapy) means the postmenopausal therapy contains only a form of **estrogen**.

The advantages of long-term replacement of estradiol over-whelmingly outweigh the risks and solve issues in areas of the body you may not realize are related to estrogen and menopause.

- Cardiovascular disease is the number one cause of death in women. Estrogen decreases the risk of heart disease by lowering cholesterol, increasing the level of protective HDL cholesterol, and reducing the inflammation that increases cholesterol's ability to deposit in blood vessels. It follows that estrogen protects us against heart attack and stroke, as both are dependent on atherosclerosis of the vessels (hardening of the arteries) to occur.

- Diabetes and insulin resistance (hypoglycemia) decrease when estradiol is replaced by decreasing abdominal fat and insulin resistance. The same results are not seen with HRT (estrogen plus progestin), as progestins counteract the effects of estrogen.

- Weight gain and obesity are prevented by replacing testosterone and ERT as well. Kathy's findings, from the data on the women who come to her office, confirm the belief that weight loss is assisted by replacing bio-identical testosterone and estradiol.

- Osteoporosis and vertebral fractures occur rapidly after estradiol drops at menopause. These changes occur almost entirely in the first five years after menopause. Early intervention can prevent fractures from estrogen deprivation in the vertebral disks. Both estradiol and testosterone stimulate the growth of bone as well as the absorption of calcium from the GI tract. Both hormones perform more efficiently than bisphosphonates, like Fosamax, and make thicker bones less likely to fracture.

- Researchers from SUNY at Stony Brook found that estradiol even protects lungs from damage. Under low-oxygen environments resulting from disease or environmental toxins, estrogenized guinea pigs had less pulmonary damage. These findings are thought to be applicable to humans.

- HRT may help decrease the risk for developing colon cancer. Studies of this disease have been done in regard to estrogen replacement, and in 1998 the Heart and Estrogen/progestin Replacement Study (HERS) found that there were fewer cases of colon cancer in patients on estradiol or HRT. This is thought to result from the effect of estrogen suppressing bile acid production that sometimes promotes colon cancer, and progesterone suppressing the speed of growth of cells in the colon.

- Macular degeneration, or vision loss, is another disease of aging, but it is also one of the diseases that can be prevented by replacing estrogen. Estrogen treats the inflammation and prevents the damage that leads to macular degeneration.

Estradiol Replacement and Alzheimer's and Other Dementias

Alzheimer's is one of the most feared of diseases and one of the most responsive to estrogen replacement, so let's examine it in a little more depth. Loss of memory at menopause is one of the early warning signs that you need your hormones replaced and, more important, that long-term deprivation may cause worsening memory loss and, finally, dementia. This is one of the most compelling reasons to replace estradiol.

In the Seattle Study, reported in the January 2013 *Journal of Menopause*, 62 percent of midlife women complained of difficulty concentrating, poor recall of names and words, forgetfulness of events, disorganized thought, and loss of work efficiency. These symptoms represent the loss of connection of neurons and the slowing of the thought process that comes with loss of testosterone and estradiol. Estradiol stimulates the growth of neuronal extension and branching. It also scavenges damaged cells in the brain, preventing the formation of neurons with the development of plaque that causes Alzheimer's disease.

Research on Alzheimer's disease has found that the female brain actually shrinks when it is not exposed to estrogen. In a 2006 study, MRIs were used to measure the brain volume of women taking ERT compared to women not taking estrogen. The subsequent measures of brain gray matter, brain volume, and cognitive tests were all greater in women who replaced estradiol.

If your family history includes Alzheimer's or dementia, long-term studies have shown that patients who replace estradiol in the ten years after menopause delay the occurrence of Alzheimer's disease and other dementias by ten years. This is the only known "prevention" for Alzheimer's and dementia. Replacing estradiol and testosterone can repair and replace neurons that have undergone the aging process. Memory responds quickly, and neurotransmitters are recovered for normal neurologic function soon after replacement begins in the first ten years after menopause or TDS.

When the diseases that result from estrogen loss are viewed as a group, the argument to replace estrogen as well as testosterone is overwhelmingly made by preventive effectiveness alone. Treatment options are the next step in a choice for or against estrogen and HRT replacement.

TREATMENT CHOICES FOR MENOPAUSE

When considering treatment for the symptoms of menopause, it's important to know what your choices are and the differences among treatment options. Your doctor may treat menopause by ordering a "one size fits all" prescription, or order lab tests, or choose a customized treatment.

Medicine uses abbreviations when describing treatments or conditions, and it is important to properly know what they are talking about to discuss your problems. In the case of hormone replacement, the terms ERT and HRT represent two types of treatments that can be selected to treat women with menopausal symptoms. ERT, estrogen replacement therapy, literally means replacing only estrogen to treat menopausal symptoms. ERT also indicates a category of prescription drugs consisting of estrogenlike medications given without a progestin. Only women without a uterus can take estrogenlike replacement alone, unless they are using small doses of estrogen applied to the vagina, where absorption is minimal. Estrogen alone, when given systemically without progestin or progesterone, can stimulate uterine bleeding if a uterus is present. When given to a patient with a uterus, ERT can also cause uterine cancer if taken over a long-term period.

The H in HRT does not stand for any hormone in the body, as there are many, but by agreement among researchers, specifically relates to this combination of estrogen and progestin. (It may be confusing, but using H to mean both estrogen and progestin makes it simpler for research notations.)

When women speak with their doctors, they're told that HRT refers *only* to estrogen and progestin. This is currently the common usage. However, HRT should also include the replacement of testosterone. When TDS is accepted, that will be the new standard.

The estrogen in the definition can be any form of estrogen: for example, Premarin, Ogen, or estradiol. Progestin means any drug that is progesteronelike and that prevents the buildup of the lining of the uterus.

HRT combination replacement is given to women with a uterus to both replace estrogen and treat symptoms of menopause while also protecting the uterus from bleeding and cancer. There is a drawback to using HRT with a progestin instead of bio-identical progesterone. Progestins are quickly changed in the liver into estrone and undesirable androgens that both stimulate breast tissue and may stimulate the growth of a breast cancer.

Synthetic HRT (estrogen plus progestin) and ERT (estrogen alone) delivery systems divided by type of therapy: Local application is for absorption into the skin to improve the quality of that area without systemic absorption. Systemic delivery is meant to supply the whole body.

Hormone Options		
Delivery System	**Type of Therapy**	**Traditional Synthetic Hormones**
Vaginal estrogen	Local therapy for dry vagina and painful intercourse	Premarin vaginal cream, Estrace vaginal cream, Vagifem vaginal tablets
Synthetic estrogen transdermal patch	Systemic therapy	Climara patch, Vivelle patch, CombiPatch, Climara Pro patch
Synthetic oral estrogen only pills	Systemic therapy	Premarin, Estrace, Ogen, generic estradiol
Synthetic estrogen and progestin oral HRT	Systemic therapy	Prempro, Femhrt

The Current Mainstream Medical Treatment for Menopause

For most menopausal women, doctors write a prescription for HRT, a combination of a synthetic estrogen and progestin. The purpose is to treat the symptoms of menopause with the necessary estrogen and prevent a postmenopausal uterus from bleeding by using progestin. Progestins provide protection for the uterine lining. These HRT prescriptions act like the hormones you made in your ovaries but are not bio-identical. They are effective for decreasing the symptoms of menopause but have many side effects. This is because they break down in the stomach and liver into chemicals that are not like any hormone that your body made in youth. This breakdown occurs before the hormones do any work in your body, so you are exposed to the detrimental metabolites that cause side effects, not the true, natural hormone that could provide many benefits. These side effects can include weight gain, breast tenderness and growth, increased clotting risk, increased risk of liver tumors (with oral hormones), uterine bleeding, fibroid growth, decreased active forms of thyroid and testosterone hormones, and suppression of sex drive.

Conversely, bio-identical hormones resemble the hormones your body made earlier in life and act like the native hormones when they are absorbed. Thus they cause fewer side effects than synthetic hormones and are more effective in re-creating the youthful hormone environment. Bio-identical hormones cannot tolerate the acid-rich environment of the stomach, so they must be given in nonoral forms in order for the body to metabolize them properly.

Synthetic hormones create a whole host of side effects for most women and fewer benefits when compared to bio-identical hormone replacement. In 2002 the WHI study put an end to pharmaceutical companies' creation of new synthetic estrogens and progestins for menopause because of gross misinterpretation of the study in the headlines.

Since 2001 birth control pills have been approved by the FDA for menopause HRT in nonsmokers over age 35. Doctors who are comfortable with them for menopause continue prescribing them as their patients transition from fertility to menopause without changing prescriptions. Unfortunately, these pills contain such a low dose of estrogen that most of the protective effects of estrogen after menopause (such as prevention of heart disease, Alzheimer's disease, and osteoporosis) are lost. This option is convenient for the doctor because patients continue the same medication without any adjustment problems, such as vaginal bleeding, that are sometimes seen as they change types of hormone replacement. But it offers minimal relief of symptoms of aging and menopause, and it does not provide the essential hormone, testosterone. Therefore, women who choose birth control pills for their postmenopausal replacement do not enjoy the benefits of replacing estrogen, testosterone, and when needed progesterone, that we have been discussing throughout this book.

Synthetic Nonoral Hormone Replacement for Menopause
Birth control patch (Ortho Evra)
Vaginal birth control ring (NuvaRing)
Hormone replacement patch (Climara, Climara Pro, Vivelle, and CombiPatch)
Estrogen replacement estrogen ring (Estring)
Transdermal cream (Estrasorb, Elestra)

There are many varieties of hormone replacement available to your gynecologist for the treatment of symptoms of menopause. The downside of some of these medications is that they can be synthetic, and therefore inactivate free testosterone by binding it with SHBG (sex hormone binding globulin). The suppression of testosterone in turn causes undesirable side effects such as belly fat, depression, insulin resistance, and decreased libido. Out of the group of synthetic HRTs your doctor may give you, the best are non-oral: they avoid the first-pass effect, which impacts their absorption process in the body. Synthetic estrogen replacement is the riskiest and the least effective and is translated into undesirable by-products by the first-pass effect.

Every synthetic oral HRT has the same issues:

- It must be taken every day or those patients with a uterus will bleed.
- It *suppresses* testosterone and *increases* estrone.
- It does not bring FSH back to premenopausal levels.
- It brings estrogen levels up and down over a 24-hour period, causing irritability and moodiness.

Oral HRT also carries a host of warnings:

- It is not always absorbed in patients taking antacids and ulcer medications.
- It cannot be taken if you have liver disease.

- It cannot be taken by patients with history of blood clots because it increases clotting factors.

- It increases sex hormone binding globulin (SHBG) and inactivates testosterone, reducing the benefits of any testosterone replacement.

- It causes raised blood pressure, weight gain, increased abdominal circumference, decreased muscle mass, water retention, and increased chances of getting prediabetes and diabetes, along with general fatigue.

Transdermal HRT includes creams, patches, gels, and vaginal tablets. This form of estrogen replacement has fewer side effects than oral HRT and all birth control pills. With transdermal HRT, there is less suppression of testosterone and less estrone production and therefore less risk of breast cancer and blood clots. The latest American Congress of Obstetricians and Gynecologists guidelines document that nonoral estrogen replacement does not increase the risk of recurrent deep venous thrombosis (DVT), blood clots. However, there is a huge drawback to many of the transdermal delivery systems. The gels and creams may have to be dosed anywhere from 1 to 3 times a day. Patches have the advantage of being dosed one to two times a week. Even though these transdermal preparations are safe, they do not provide protection from postmenopausal bleeding, which is the risk of taking any type of estrogen if you have a uterus.

Replacing hormones through the skin has an added drawback for women over 65. Advanced age is often accompanied by poor circulation to the skin; as a result transdermal hormones are poorly absorbed. The most common complaints about patches are that they cause a rash and itching and come off easily before they are scheduled to. Creams are really inconvenient because they have a short duration and must be applied several times a day, and are not absorbed in a uniform fashion from day to day, which causes moodiness.

Kathy's biggest criticism of traditional synthetic hormone therapy in any type of delivery system is that the recommended doses are too low to treat all the symptoms of menopause, as evidenced by the fact that recommended doses do not suppress FSH to premenopausal levels. In addition, recommendations for HRT completely leave testosterone out of the guidelines. This may be because there are no nonoral forms of testosterone approved by the FDA. So traditional recommended treatment attends to the symptoms of loss of estradiol such as hot flashes, dry vagina, and dry skin but ignores symptoms of lack of testosterone such as loss of libido, memory, and muscle mass.

In general, the prescriptions that are currently written by OB/GYNs and family-practice doctors have the advantage of being easy to fill at any pharmacy and are covered by insurance.

We've seen the advantages and disadvantages of the synthetic hormone replacement therapies currently used by OB/GYNs. Now we want to tell you about bio-identical therapies.

THE NEW WAY TO TREAT MENOPAUSE: BIO-IDENTICAL HORMONE THERAPY

Bio-identical hormones include estradiol, progesterone, and testosterone. There are a number of delivery options: oral, transdermal (through the skin), sublingual (under the tongue), buccal (absorbed through the cheek), vaginal, transdermal skin creams and gels, intramuscular (shots), and subcutaneous pellets (inserted into the fat of the hip to dissolve over a period of four to six months). We will discuss this further in Chapter 9.

Most OB/GYNs are not trained in bio-identical hormone prescription and management. They are often reluctant to write the prescription because they don't know how to adjust the therapy. They also have little experience with compounding pharmacies, so they don't know how to dose or write the compounded prescriptions.

As we learned in Chapter 2, the BNDD and the FDA regulate the production and use of bio-identical hormones; but they do not "approve" them, even though bio-identical hormones are superior and have demonstrated better results. (And as you now know, doctors use many other off-label drugs—those prescribed for purposes other than uses approved by the FDA—so that should not influence their decision.)

If you want to try bio-identical hormones, ask your doctor if she prescribes them for menopause. Let your doctor know that you want this type of therapy and that you are willing to pay for it out of pocket if need be. If she doesn't prescribe them, ask for a referral to a hormone specialist. If that is not possible in your area, ask a pharmacist at a compounding pharmacy for the name of a doctor who prescribes compounded bio-identical hormone therapy. (Use the key words "compounding pharmacy" and "bio-identical therapy" in your search engine.)

Bio-identical Hormonal Delivery Systems

The most important thing to know about bio-identical hormones is that the way they are delivered is the key to managing their side effects. Most synthetic hormones have one or two delivery methods (oral or patches); but bio-identicals offer multiple choices, and it is the delivery system that makes the difference in safety, effectiveness, and side effects. Oral hormones have a first-pass effect through the liver that decomposes them into a variety of components that cause side effects. Transdermal, sublingual, and vaginal hormones are more like our own hormones, but they still change chemical composition as they penetrate the skin or mucosa of the vagina. The change causes estradiol and testosterone to metabolize into estrone, the form of estrogen that causes multiple side effects. The best delivery system for estradiol and testosterone is one that delivers both hormones directly to the bloodstream, replicating the hormones secreted by the ovary when you were younger. Pure hormones delivered to the bloodstream are the most physiologic forms and allow women to feel just like they did when they were premenopausal.

After menopause the only estradiol and testosterone replacement that re-creates the normal estradiol-to-estrone relationship is bio-identical estradiol and testosterone pellets.

Estrogen Source	Estradiol:Estrone
Youthful ovary	2:1
Oral ERT pills	1:10
Patch	1:5
Gel	1:2
Bio-identical vaginal tablets	1:1
Bio-identical pellets E+T	2:1

Estradiol pellets placed under the skin are the best delivery method for resolving symptoms and maintaining a premenopausal-like biologic environment with a 2:1 ratio of estradiol to estrone. Estradiol and testosterone pellets are placed beneath the skin (after making a small incision) and deliver the hormones to the bloodstream as a time-release system. They dissolve slowly in the fat of the hip where they are placed, as you need them. Patients who receive replacement hormones with pellets are given a "reservoir" of hormones that can be accessed on demand when the body needs them.

Women whose symptoms are not alleviated by over-the-counter medications or traditional hormone therapy make some of the best bio-identical hormone pellet candidates. One of the symptoms of high estrogen levels is uterine bleeding. Our goal is to get patients back to the balance they enjoyed in their 30s, and we do *not* believe that having a period during the menopausal years is necessary or even helpful on a monthly basis. However, when we replace estradiol and give you sublingual or buccal progesterone, the uterus is stimulated and sometime bleeds. This is the most difficult problem we encounter, yet it is not life threatening.

There are ways to treat this symptom. First, we balance the estradiol with testosterone pellets and sublingual or pellet progesterone. Arimidex (an aromatase blocker) can be prescribed to shrink fibroids and stop bleeding from them. If hormonal interventions don't work, we employ surgical methods to stop uterine bleeding, such as D&C (dilation and curettage), THERMACHOICE uterine ablation, hysteroscopic surgery, and even hysterectomy. Finally, monitoring your hormone blood levels and, when indicated, changing the dose of the next pellet insertion or next dose of bio-identical hormone are the most effective practices.

There are some alternate therapies to hormonal treatment for menopause. For example, the antidepressant Effexor can be used to eliminate hot flashes, but no other symptoms of menopause. Estroven, an OTC, soy-based herbal supplement, works for mild hot flashes but not for the whole host of symptoms experienced during menopause. Some women have tried acupuncture or massage for relief of minimal symptoms. When you experiment with these various options, you must ask yourself: *Do these efforts bring enough relief for my symptoms? Am I bringing enough resources to fight the problem?*

For patients who want relief from all of their symptoms, bio-identical estrogen and testosterone, with or without bio-identical progesterone, in a nonoral delivery system is our recommended treatment for menopause. It is also the safest treatment. Vaginal preparations are effective, but pellet subcutaneous implants are ideal because they are the most successful. Ninety-five percent of the time, they restore women to their premenopausal selves.

IF YOU CANNOT TAKE ESTROGENS

Typically, all medications and OTC remedies have some side effects and limitations, so certain patients cannot take them. Those who cannot take estrogen of any kind include patients with estrogen-receptor-positive breast cancers and those who have had a spontaneous blood clot (DVT) in the past. These two conditions are referred to as "contraindications." Fortunately, there's an alternative to estrogen that resolves most symptoms of estrogen deficit—testosterone.

Testosterone is an excellent substitute for estradiol in women who cannot take estradiol after menopause. Often there is a

crossover between the response to symptoms of estradiol and testosterone deficiency. Because they both lock on to the same receptor
site on cells, we can sometimes treat the symptoms of estrogen deficiency effectively with testosterone. Because testosterone has fewer
side effects and can be taken in the face of some diseases where
estradiol is risky, we can use testosterone to treat hot flashes, depression, anxiety, vaginal dryness, and fatigue, even in the absence
of estradiol. This is most effectively done with pellets, but other
nonoral forms can be used as well.

High Risk Candidates for Estradiol Replacement

For menopausal patients who have had a blood clot (DVT) and
would like to take estradiol in addition to testosterone, we offer a
blood test—a blood panel that tests for genetic markers to predict
whether they have the genetic risk for developing a blood clot
again. If a patient is positive for some of these tests, we avoid estradiol replacement. In the case of other positive genetic markers, we
can normalize the risk by treating with folic acid in large doses,
daily low-dose aspirin, and estradiol, without increasing risk of
clotting. Alternately, if all your genetic markers are negative, you
are not at increased risk for future blood clots and therefore are no
more likely than anyone else to get a second blood clot, on or off
estrogen. The negative test allows us to use estradiol even in the
case of a history of DVT and pulmonary embolism.

The Blood Clot Risk Panel

- Antiphospholipid antibodies positive increase risk
- Antithrombin III—deficiency increases risk
- Factor V Leiden mutation—increases risk seven times
- Homocysteine elevation increases risk of blood clots
- MTHFR—if two positive genes (homozygous),
  increased risk of clotting

- Protein C—deficiency causes clotting
- Protein S—deficiency increases risk
- Prothrombin G20210A mutation

To see if you have a high genetic risk of getting a recurrent blood clot, you can have the high-risk blood panel drawn.

Of course, anyone can have a DVT without any of these risk factors, but you are less likely to repeat the problem, even on replacement estrogen, if your blood tests are negative. Smoking and inactivity can increase the risk of blood clots under any circumstances, with or without genetic risk or estradiol replacement. Testosterone does not increase the risk of blood clot formation.

Benefits of Estradiol Replacement

If you're a good candidate for estrogen, the benefits of estradiol replacement are many. By replacing estradiol in the safest way, you can avoid many diseases of old age and get your quality of life back with little risk. To decide whether this is right for you, you must look at the risks and benefits of taking estradiol and not taking it. Following are the benefits of replacing estradiol:

- Decreases obesity
- Decreases risk of Alzheimer's disease
- Improves arthritis
- Improves bone density better than Fosamax-like drugs
- Improves irritable bladder; prevents urinary tract infections
- Improves sight and slows aging
- Improves sleep
- Improves stress incontinence
- Prevents diabetes
- Prevents heart disease
- Prevents macular degeneration, loss of vision

- Thickens vaginal and pelvic tissue for more comfortable sex

The risks of replacing estradiol depend on the *type of estrogen* you choose. The risks of taking any type of estradiol include:

- Growth of fibroids
- Swelling
- Uterine cancer (only if no progesterone is taken)
- Vaginal bleeding

Oral forms of estradiol replacement can lead to increasing growth rates in existing breast cancer, but they do not *cause* breast cancer. Nonoral estradiol does not increase the risk of breast cancer or DVT. Both oral and nonoral forms can increase the risk of developing the medical problems listed above, but doctors have methods of surveillance so the problems can be caught in a timely fashion. The critical difference would be if there is an untreated breast cancer. Breast cancer cells act differently from normal breast cells, so we withhold estrogen until the cancer is treated, then reevaluate. Testosterone can still be given to reduce symptoms.

Many diseases can be prevented through estradiol replacement, but every woman has the choice to take replacement hormones or not. For those women with symptoms of estradiol deprivation, the choice to take estradiol is easier than for those without current symptoms. Other women who do not have symptoms of menopause have a more difficult time deciding to take replacement hormones in any form to prevent future illness because they are not bothered by things like persistent hot flashes.

Now that you have read all the information regarding progesterone and estrogen, it is time to consider your options. In Part III, we will guide you through these decisions. We'll look at the different ways you can be treated, financial costs, and the risks and benefits. Once you have gone through this process, you'll be able to take this information to your physician, discuss what you have learned, and figure out what's best for you.

PART III

MOVING FORWARD

CHAPTER 8

THE RISKS
AND BENEFITS
OF REPLACING
TESTOSTERONE,
ESTROGEN, OR
PROGESTERONE

Before you make a choice between taking a replacement hormone or not, you must go through the decision-making process. This boils down to looking at each hormone and weighing its pros and cons. Some will be more important than others to you depending on your personal values, medical and family history, and other factors. Remember: this is all about *you,* so please consider all of the information as it pertains to you. As you go, keep track of which benefits outweigh the risks of taking a certain hormone and which ones you have questions about. If your belief is that you will never replace your hormones, remember there is a risk to not replacing them, as well.

We'll begin by defining some of the terms often used in medicine that you will find throughout this chapter. We want you to be comfortable with this terminology so you can concentrate on making the best decision for your health.

A *side effect* is an unwanted or unintended effect of a medical therapy that is unhealthy or undesirable. For example, facial hair growth on a woman taking testosterone is an undesired outcome of replacing that hormone; however, it is not dangerous or harmful, just a nuisance. We have found that many such side effects are easily and inexpensively treated or prevented.

A *contraindication* is a preexisting medical condition or a medication already being taken by the patient that may cause more harm than good if the medical treatment or replacement of a hormone is undertaken. For men, an example of a contraindication to testosterone is the presence of active prostate cancer.

Risk is a little more complicated to define. One way to define a risk when evaluating a medical decision is to remember that we are talking about the risk of *one person* out of a *group of people* getting a side effect or no effect from any medical treatment. The risk in hormone replacement is that the treatment may not work for you even though it works for others, or it may cause a side effect for you that it does not cause for everyone taking the same treatment. In order to make a good decision, you have to be aware of the risks of all known unintended outcomes as you consider what to do. If the chances of a specific risk is 1 out of 10,000, then the chance of your getting by without a specific problem is 9,999 of 10,000. This is a realistic way to calculate the odds. I have always believed that a risk is a negative outcome to be considered seriously, even if the risk is low. When you embark on any treatment, if the 1 in 10,000 turns out to be *you*, it is 100 percent your problem.

Choosing not to have hormone replacement therapy also carries risks. Those who choose to do nothing should ask themselves, "What is the risk of doing nothing?" There are always risks that accompany inaction. For example, if I start to run a red light and hit the brakes, I have a chance of jostling my passengers or having the car bump into me from behind. That is the risk of hitting the brakes. The risk of not hitting the brakes (doing nothing) is that the cross traffic that is entering the intersection will crash into my car and injure my passengers and me. That, most would agree, is a greater risk. This is an unconscious process we all do daily, so let's use the same process to decide on a treatment plan.

We will list the risks and benefits of every hormone and delivery system, as well as the qualities of bio-identical hormones versus corresponding synthetic hormones. Because TDS is the core of this book, we will start with the first hormone you may need to replace, testosterone.

BENEFITS OF TESTOSTERONE REPLACEMENT

Testosterone is both the least risky and most beneficial hormone to replace in women as long as the delivery method is chosen carefully. Consequently, it is the first hormone most women need and seek to replace.

The benefits of testosterone are many and the symptoms of TDS are also multiple. We have gone over the symptoms of TDS in detail, so you should be very familiar with what happens without testosterone. The benefits are the flip side of TDS: increased energy, restorative sleep, loss of fat, leanness, balanced temperament, excellent memory, freedom from joint and muscular pain, physical stamina, sense of well-being, sex drive and orgasms, relief from migraine headaches, skin tone, motivation or "mojo," defined muscles and muscle strength, balanced mood . . . the list goes on and on. There is a lot of benefit from just one hormone.

Benefits can also include decreasing the number and cost of the prescriptions you take. As we discovered in Chapter 6, testosterone replacement can help prevent or delay diseases like osteoporosis, Alzheimer's disease, heart disease, stroke, obesity, diabetes, and frailty that leads to nursing home life. You should look at your family history of diseases to see if any of the illnesses testosterone prevents run in your family. If they do, testosterone replacement may help you avoid them in the future.

RISKS, COSTS, AND EFFECTIVENESS OF ALL TYPES OF TESTOSTERONE REPLACEMENT

Most of the risks involved in taking testosterone as pellets are cosmetic and minor, if you get them at all. The only life-threatening testosterone replacement is an oral, synthetic testosterone, Estratest, and these dangers do not apply to the other forms of testosterone. Risks of all types of testosterone include:

- Facial hair growth
- Increased pubic and body hair
- Lowered pitch of the voice
- Increased muscle mass
- Increased oil production in the skin
- Acne
- Temporary clitoral enlargement
- Temporary hypersexuality
- Thinning of hair on head
- Vulvar swelling and itching
- Liver tumors

The majority of these risks are not life threatening or even medically dangerous, and are mostly temporary, preventable, or treatable. Most women only get fuzzy facial hair on their upper lip and never encounter the remainder of these side effects.

It's important to distinguish the specific risks of bio-identical and synthetic testosterone delivery systems. The comparison that begins on the following page should help in deciding what to discuss with your doctor. The first replacement is synthetic, and it is the only testosterone replacement approved by the FDA for women. We've included it so you can compare the risks with the rest of the bio-identical forms of testosterone replacement.

- **Estratest**—synthetic oral combination of testosterone and estrogen:

  Risks: Liver hepatomas (i.e., tumors on the liver from direct exposure to oral testosterone), weight gain, breast tenderness, blood clots, anger and aggression, increase in blood lipids
  Relief of symptoms: Moderate for all symptoms other than hot flashes
  Benefits: Once-daily dosing, covered by insurance
  Cost: Co-pay
  Insurance: Covered by most plans

- **Oral bio-identical testosterone:**

  Risks: Weight gain, breast tenderness and pain, breast enlargement, increased estrone production, anger and aggression, elevated blood lipids, abundant facial hair, and rare cases of liver hepatomas
  Relief of symptoms: Moderate for all symptoms other than hot flashes
  Benefits: Once-daily dosing, good absorption, stable blood levels, and bio-identical
  Cost: $90 to $100/month
  Insurance: May not be covered

- **Bio-identical testosterone vaginal tabs and vaginal creams:**

  Risks: Weight gain, breast tenderness, moderate estrone production, and variable blood levels of testosterone that do not reflect symptom resolution.
  Relief of symptoms: Good relief of some symptoms but has variable absorption (absorption rates differ as metabolism differs among women by age, activity, and weight levels). Blood levels are constantly variable, and it is very hard to maintain stable blood levels or relief of symptoms. No increased libido and mood; does not make an effective amount of free testosterone necessary to cross to the brain; poor absorption in menopausal woman with vaginal atrophy; messy.
  Benefits: Dosing once per day but inconsistent absorption; bio-identical; decreases blood lipids

Cost: $100 to $200/month
Insurance: Not covered

- **Bio-identical testosterone sublingual (under the tongue) tablet:**

   Risks: Very rarely is absorbed in measurable amounts; unpleasant taste
   Relief of symptoms: Rarely produces a significant blood level; minimal relief of symptoms; minimal and inconsistent benefit
   Benefits: Dosing once or twice per day; bio-identical
   Cost: $90 to $125/month
   Insurance: Not covered

- **Bio-identical testosterone transdermal cream and gel:**

   Risks: Poor absorption with variable blood levels depending on the blood flow to the skin and varies with temperature (poor absorption when weather is cold); transferrable to children and spouse through body contact; increases local hair production so areas of application grow unusual hair patches; allergies; excessive hair loss; weight gain and swelling; mood swings occur as doses go up and down throughout the day
   Relief of symptoms: Minimal symptom relief, but is more effective for local reduction of vaginal dryness and vulvar atrophy; does not always increase libido and mood because it does not make an effective amount of free testosterone necessary to cross to the brain
   Benefits: Dosing one to four times a day; fair absorption; bio-identical; patient can control dosing
   Cost: $100 to $200/month
   Insurance: Not covered

- **Synthetic testosterone patch:**

   Risks: Increased breast stimulation and tenderness, weight gain, facial hair, cholesterol, and blood lipids

Relief of symptoms: Good blood level; testosterone is well absorbed and can achieve the blood level necessary to resolve the presenting symptoms; moderate relief of symptoms

Benefits: Dosing once a day; effective for some TDS symptoms

Cost: Unknown

Insurance: Covered by some plans

- **Testosterone cypionate intramuscular injection:**

  Risks: Increase in weight and belly fat; heavy facial hair; hair loss; increased cholesterol and blood lipids. Short-term use has lower risks than long-term use.

  Relief of symptoms: Good blood level and moderate to complete relief of symptoms. Blood levels peak two weeks after injection and are suboptimal early and late in dosing cycle.

  Benefits: Dosing once a month with monthly doctor's office visits; effective for most TDS symptoms

  Cost: $50/month plus office visit co-pay = approximately $100/month

  Insurance: Covered by some plans

- **Bio-identical testosterone pellets subdermal (time-release delivery):**

  Risks: Insertion process can lead to infection, expulsion (pellets come out), bleeding, or bruising during insertion.

  Relief of symptoms: Excellent; consistent blood level; complete relief of symptoms for four to six months

  Benefits: Bio-identical; dosing is convenient once every four to six months; decreases estrone, cholesterol, and CRP (inflammation); suppresses estrone production and decreases risk of breast cancer; excellent muscle mass and improves growth hormone; activates fat loss; brings back excellent libido and orgasms; all symptoms of TDS are treated

  Cost: $120/month

  Insurance: Not covered

Most medical therapy is aimed at achieving the same hormonal environment that we had when we were young and healthy. However, testosterone therapy goals must be higher than are found in normal 20- to 30-year-old women for several reasons. Post-TDS women require a higher level of free testosterone than they did when they were young because their receptor sites decrease in number with age and estradiol competes with testosterone for the same receptor sites.

The outcome is that the "normal" we look for to compare our patients to young, healthy levels before replacement is not the same "normal" we shoot for after treatment. Free testosterone in a blood test must be 20 to 40 pg/dl to achieve normal hormonal balance and the relief of TDS symptoms. Different normals are identified when we are diagnosing than when we are replacing. Because everyone's metabolism is unique to them, we have to find the operative level for each patient while remembering that after menopause, they need more than they did before. Free testosterone is the only testosterone that penetrates the blood-brain barrier and enters the brain.

Each type of testosterone requires a different blood level that parallels the resolution of the symptoms of TDS. For instance, blood levels found in women using vaginal testosterone suppositories or tablets are sometimes in the thousands without relief of symptoms, while the level of testosterone needed for symptom resolution in testosterone pellets is in the 30s to 40s. The levels are so variable for each type of testosterone that it is important to see a doctor who is familiar with the goal of therapy for various kinds of testosterone to ensure your levels are monitored accurately.

Some forms of testosterone replacement are not easily managed by measuring blood levels because symptoms do not correlate with blood levels at all. No one has investigated this unusual finding. Kathy does not recommend these forms of treatment because of the lack of symptom correlation. Her findings with vaginal testosterone (unreliable blood levels) compared to subcutaneous pellet testosterone replacement (very predictive of symptoms) are an example of this difference.

Testosterone and Breast Cancer

Many women are fearful of replacing their testosterone because they fear breast cancer. What they do not know is that testosterone replacement can help reduce the risk of getting breast cancer as well as decrease the risk of reoccurrence of a previous breast cancer. Their fear comes from an underlying public ignorance of what testosterone does in the body; it is actually protective against many types of cancer. Most breast oncologists understand the effectiveness of testosterone when treating menopausal symptoms and approve testosterone replacements for their breast-cancer patients.

How Does Testosterone Protect Against Breast Cancer?

- Stimulates T cell production and activity (T cells kill cancer cells)

- Stimulates the whole immune system to fight cancer cells

- Competes with estrogen for breast cells and suppresses breast growth and activity

Testosterone is currently given to HIV-positive patients to treat and suppress their cancers, treat depression, and build muscle and bone. It is the original immune stimulant and is one of the hormones that keeps us from getting cancers and immune illnesses when we are young.

If you want to decrease your risk of breast cancer, or if you have a strong family history and want to delay the onset of a breast cancer, replace testosterone and add supplements that help fight cancer. Vitamins act as catalysts to most of the chemical reactions in the body, so for a woman to build muscle, replace cells in her bone marrow, build bone, and digest food in addition to millions of microscopic enzyme reactions, she needs every essential vitamin and mineral supplied in her diet. Frequent deficiencies found in the United States are vitamins D, C, and A, iodine, and the minerals calcium and magnesium. Optimal nutrition and the provision of every essential vitamin and mineral act to repair damaged cells and stimulate immune system activity. There is one supplement made of cauliflower and broccoli called DIM (diindolylmethane) that performs somewhat like the drug Arimidex, an aromatase inhibitor. This supplement decreases estrone, the estrogen that is thought to be the culprit that stimulates breast cancer cells. Both DIM and Arimidex work by blocking an enzyme reaction that converts testosterone into estrone. DIM decreases the amount of estrone in the body and in the breast, which decreases breast size, overall body fat, and breast cell turnover. Both DIM and Arimidex decrease the risk that a cell in the breast can become cancerous. Arimidex is currently used to prevent and treat estrogen-receptor-positive breast cancer by decreasing estrone. It is now replacing the drug tamoxifen.

The best prevention of recurrent breast cancer was found to be a combination of bio-identical testosterone pellets plus Arimidex. The results of a five-year study of this combination was released in 2012. The study found that the combination prevented recurrence of breast cancer over a period of five years in women who had survived breast cancer, as well as to suppress symptoms of menopause (without estrogen) and improve libido and energy. This outcome is most likely due to testosterone's stimulatory effect on the immune system as well as reduction of estrone.

WHO CAN'T TAKE TESTOSTERONE REPLACEMENT?

Some individuals have an existing medical problem, or have not finished child bearing, or are among those who chose not to take permanent birth control. These patients will need to focus on symptomatic treatments rather than seek correction of their hormone imbalances.

For any of the following issues, testosterone replacement is not generally recommended, although many women who have these contraindications can take certain types of testosterone if they have procedures such as an intrauterine device (IUD) for birth control or giving blood two to three times a year to decrease red blood counts.

- Chronic liver disease such as hepatitis that impairs liver function and metabolism of testosterone by-products
- Liver tumors (oral contraindicated only)
- High concentration of platelets
- High concentration of red blood cells (polycythemia)
- Premenopausal fertility without permanent birth control

For women without these complications, evaluating the risks and benefits of testosterone replacement in general, and specifically each type of testosterone replacement, will provide the most usable information upon which to base a decision.

Looking at the Costs for Testosterone Replacement

Because insurance companies have not yet recognized testosterone for women as a necessary treatment, they do not cover it. This means that testosterone treatments must be paid for out of pocket, but the benefits—as they say in the credit card commercials—are *priceless!* How much would you pay in order to walk, run, play, and make love the way you did when you were 35? If you have lost these abilities, you know you would pay almost anything to get them back. The cost is relative and varies by parts of the country and types of testosterone replacement. We will review the average costs of treatment, but keep in mind the monetary cost of not taking testosterone. How will the deterioration of muscles and bones that accompanies aging in the absence of testosterone affect your cost of living?

For the majority of women, choosing not to replace testosterone will result in a large percentage of their retirement income being spent on multiple medications (one for each symptom), co-pays, doctors' appointments, and surgery. If your method of aging is to use all the vitamins and supplements available, weight loss plans, and exercise schemes to build muscle without the help of testosterone, you can end up spending a large percentage of your income on alternative therapies and/or nursing facilities in the distant future.

If these future health maladies have not made you get out your calculator, consider the work environment and how important it is for you to look and act youthful to compete in the job market. How can you compete with younger, more vibrant employees for your job if your motivation is gone, you aren't thinking clearly, you are starting to make mistakes, and you are not able to meet deadlines?

And those are only the short-term considerations! As you have learned, the costs of *not* taking testosterone are longer term and extremely expensive. The cascade of problems stemming from loss of testosterone with age is extensive—and very expensive to treat.

It is clear that in terms of improving quality of life and preventing the misery of multiple illnesses in the future, testosterone can be a godsend. If the cost of therapy is the hurdle that is the most difficult for you, sit down with a pencil and paper and consider the costs you are already incurring for multiple medicines, multiple doctor visits to various medical specialists, and the damage from the symptoms already listed. How do these costs compare with the cost of testosterone replacement? If you then add a basic estimate for the costs of long-term debilitating diseases, what would be the total cost of *not replacing testosterone?*

Monetarily as well as medically, the decision to take testosterone should be simple after looking at the benefits of replacement and the relief of more than a dozen symptoms of aging in the present, as well as the prevention of almost a dozen diseases in the future. This array of benefits, including recovering your sexuality, is overwhelming when compared with the most common side effect of testosterone: facial hair.

If a typical patient spends money on blood pressure medicine at an average cost of $21.50 per month, antidepressants at an average cost of $60 per month, cholesterol medications at an average cost of $40 per month, sleeping pills at $40 per month, antianxiety medications at $30 per month, and Fosamax at $60 per month (cost to the patient, not the total cost to the insurance company), she spends an average of $251.50 per month on medicines. That's more than $3,000 annually.

If she is able to drop all those costs and pay $4.60 per day on average for estrogen and testosterone replacement, her net outlay would be approximately $139.90 per month, or a total of $1,679.00 a year, for a net savings of $1,339.00 per year. This will cut her costs for medicines almost in half!

There is another issue to consider when deciding whether testosterone will work for you as it does for other people, and it includes other medications you take that might make testosterone less effective. If you are taking medications in the table below, you should make your doctor aware of this, and he or she will decide what you should do in terms of testosterone replacement or modification of the other medications.

Medications or Events That Decrease the Blood Level of Testosterone or Decrease the Effect of Testosterone
Antidepressants
Breast-feeding
Blood pressure medications
Evista
Genetic aromatase hyperactivity (converts testosterone to estrone)
Low adrenal function
Lupron therapy for endometriosis
Oral contraceptives (birth control pills)
Oral estrogens
Oral or intramuscular steroids; e.g.: Medrol dose pack, prednisone, hydrocortisone
Oral progesterone or progestins
Poor or absent ovulation
Removal of both ovaries
Tamoxifen

The decision regarding the type of testosterone to take should be a personal one based on the type of lifestyle you lead as well as your medical history, budget, and preferences for control over your dosage schedule. My advice is to choose a type of testosterone that is nonoral and bio-identical.

In Chapter 9 we will walk you through each possible means of hormone replacement to help you decide which is best for you.

BENEFITS OF ESTRADIOL REPLACEMENT

Before you dismiss estradiol replacement, let us list the pros and cons of doing this so you can decide for yourself. Remember, in Chapter 7 we explained that estradiol is the desirable, youthful estrogen women make while they are fertile. It's the hormone necessary for women's brains and bodies to develop in the womb and then to develop into women, and it benefits them in myriad ways. To review, estradiol benefits women because it:

- Improves fat distribution in the face to make women look younger
- Improves hair growth, thickness, and texture
- Improves mood
- Improves the skin of the body and vagina, making them stretchy and elastic
- Improves nail growth Produces vaginal lubrication for sex
- Increases neurotransmitters to improve memory
- Prevents Alzheimer's disease and dementia
- Prevents heart disease and increases the good cholesterol, HDL
- Prevents osteoporosis and makes better bone than current drugs can
- Prevents urinary incontinence from atrophy and irritable bladder
- *And stops hot flashes!*

From our perspective, it has all the qualities of a miracle drug for women. When combined with testosterone, estrogen acts much like a fountain of youth! But to every silver lining there is a cloud. Estrogen's safety and risk profile depend on both the kind of estrogen you take and the way you take it.

Risks of Estrogen Replacement

Most women still believe the highly publicized 2002 WHI study that said that ERT—or any "hormones" at all after menopause—cause breast cancer. This was a false conclusion that has since been proven inaccurate. In fact, a new Yale University study in 2013 claims that as many as 50,000 women may have died unnecessarily because they did not receive hormone replacement therapy. There's a possibility that the deaths between 2002 and 2012 are attributable to doctors not understanding the WHI study.

The follow-up on that study was published by independent female doctors who wrote in a headline in 2012, "Estrogen Replacement Decreases the Risk of Breast Cancer." This information comes from the WHI as well; however, it took ten years for them to straighten out the data in order to give women the right information. Sadly, it was not on any newspaper's front page; it was buried in the back. No matter where it was printed as a retraction to the earlier conclusion, it was finally a vindication for all the doctors and patients who continued to use estradiol for symptoms of menopause.

As you read this book, we would like you to forget what you have heard or read over the past 15 years that denigrates the usefulness of estrogen and instead consider the newest and best studies that offer solid information supporting the benefits of replacing estrogen after menopause.

The risks of taking an estrogen replacement are listed on the following table. These risks are divided according to whether you have had a hysterectomy or not because a uterus that is present is the biggest preventable risk of taking estradiol.

Risks and Side Effects of Estrogen Replacement	
No Hysterectomy (uterus present)	**Hysterectomy (no uterus)**
Uterine bleeding; irregular and/or heavy	
Uterine cancer	
Growth of uterine fibroids	
Breast tenderness	Breast tenderness
Breast cysts	Breast cysts
Water retention	Water retention
Blood clots & pulmonary emboli	Blood clots & pulmonary emboli

Obviously, there are more risks for women with a uterus than without. The risk of having a uterus over not having one is based on the fact that estradiol alone (without progesterone) can increase the risk of developing uterine cancer. Your risk of uterine cancer is obviously higher if you have a uterus than if you had a hysterectomy, whether you take estradiol or not!

WHO SHOULD NOT TAKE ESTROGEN?: THREE CONTRAINDICATIONS TO ERT

Before we explore the risks of each type of estrogen replacement, we must discuss the contraindications to taking any estrogen, based on your own medical history. If you have one of the three medical problems or conditions listed below, you should discuss this contraindication with your physician.

1. History of DVT or pulmonary embolism (PE). Taking estrogen may put you at risk of getting another blood clot or PE. (Nonoral estradiol does not increase this risk.)

2. History of active breast cancer with estrogen receptors. There is a risk of getting recurrent breast cancer. Women who have stage 1 breast cancer and have had a bilateral mastectomy are not at risk and can take estradiol.

3. History of endometrial (uterine lining) cancer with spread outside the uterus. There is a risk of getting recurrent uterine cancer in other areas of the abdomen. (This is not a risk for low-stage cancer.)

If you do not have any of these contraindications, estrogen replacement should definitely be a consideration for you. If you do, there are many exceptions to this rule that we will discuss.

If you have had any of these conditions in the past and are not one of the exceptions listed, prescribing estrogen for you is at the discretion of your physician. Often there are extenuating circumstances that make a case for treating women who have these contraindications, even though most women with one of these problems should not receive estrogen replacement.

WHO CAN TAKE ESTROGEN EVEN IF THEY HAVE A CONTRAINDICATION?

The standard of care is to not provide estrogen to women who have contraindications, but some patients choose to take the risk anyway. If you decide to go this route, your physician will ask you to sign a waiver releasing him or her from liability. The circumstances that allow a doctor to prescribe estrogen without a waiver and still be within the standard of care are specific to each contraindication. Attorneys would recommend that the doctor always obtain a waiver. Many doctors are willing to take the risk to treat the patient to improve their health if the patient agrees to take the risk, too. If your physician gives you his or her advice that it is dangerous for you to take estrogen, knowing the exceptions to the rule may help you discuss other options to evaluate the risk further and take preventive actions to help lower your risk so you can take estrogen in the future.

Some women also choose to take estrogen despite the risks because their quality of life is so impaired that they are willing to take the risk to regain quality of life and productivity. Women safely make these choices with a full understanding and acceptance of the risks every single day. Your physician will ask you to sign a release indemnifying him or her if you make this choice with the full knowledge of the risks involved.

Dr. Maupin's Exception to Every Rule

About seven years ago, a patient and I made an exception to the general rule about contraindications. Emily was referred to me by her son, a well-respected physician who was very concerned about his mother. She had had a blood clot on an 18-hour flight from New Zealand a number of years earlier, and her OB/GYN immediately took her off her Premarin, a popular form of estrogen. He also told her that she could never take estrogen again.

Since that day Emily had deteriorated from a funny, energetic, and lively 65-year-old to a recluse who would not leave her house. Without Premarin, she experienced extreme fatigue, incapacitating hot flashes, depression, insomnia, and agoraphobia (a fear of public places). She no longer wanted to live. Her son wanted his mother back—the robust and lively person he knew—so he pried her out of her house to consult with me.

Technically, Emily's doctor had complied with the guidelines in removing estrogen from her life, but in the process, she lost the quality of her life. My heart went out to her. As a trained OB/GYN, I had additional research at my side, and I offered her a blood panel that revealed whether a patient was at a genetic risk for recurrent blood clots. That is the real worry with estrogen and blood clots—whether someone will get another one. Medicine has many rules like these to protect us from repeating the past, but in this case I suspected Emily may *not* have been at a serious risk. The fact is that you can have a blood clot with or without a genetic defect, but those with the genetic defect are the only ones who have the risk of a recurrence when taking estrogen. The simple blood test would give us more information as to whether she possessed the genetic marker. OB/GYNs use this same test to find the reasons for recurrent miscarriages, so I was more aware of the blood panel than an internal medicine doctor might have been.

When the tests came back, Emily had only one defect out of every factor tested, and it was easily managed with an aspirin a day and folic acid. This test and intervention lowered her risk to that of a patient who had never had a blood clot. She accepted estradiol and testosterone pellets and slowly worked her way back to an active, well-traveled life!

In more than seven years of treatment, Emily has had no recurrent blood clot issues because the test correctly identified the genetic risk markers as being absent in her. Her story is one of my favorites!

Personal History of Deep Venous Thrombosis (DVT)

If you have had a blood clot in your leg or pelvis, or a pulmonary embolism, you may be at risk for another clot or embolism if you have one of the seven genetic abnormalities that put you at risk in the first place. If you don't possess any genetic mutations and your clot was just a one-time accident, your risk of a recurrent clot is the same as anyone else. If your tests are positive for mutation, you should (1) not take estrogen, (2) take estrogen with methylfolate supplements and 81 mg of aspirin a day, (3) take testosterone only, with or without aspirin and methylfolate, or use folic acid, and (4) use aspirin to counteract the hypercoagulability while you are taking estrogen. If your genetic clotting tests are negative, you have the same risk as everyone else so you may take estradiol without high-risk worries. In any case, nonoral estrogen is not contraindicated even in patients with genetic risks for blood clots.

Current or History of Estrogen-Receptor-Positive Breast Cancer

Breast cancer with estrogen-receptor-positive cells is one of the solid contraindications to taking estrogen replacement. When a breast cell becomes a cancer cell, it changes its behavior. Cancer cells lose their ability to stop multiplying and growing but may still retain their receptors to estrogen and progesterone, and these two hormones can stimulate the growth of the breast cancer cells. These receptors are usually a good sign: hormonal chemotherapy will work because the antihormone drugs will use the estrogen receptors to block and kill the cancer cells. If a breast cancer cell does not have hormone receptors for estrogen and progesterone, it means that the cancer is more aggressive and dangerous and cannot be stopped by antiestrogen chemotherapy. The one exception to this is early-stage breast cancer, which is treated by a complete bilateral mastectomy and now is approved for estrogen replacement therapy.

It is still unproven whether estrogen replacement "feeds" cancer cells for estrogen-receptive-positive cancer, causing them to grow, but it is suspected that active cancer cells are stimulated by estrogen. In this situation we offer testosterone instead of estrogen to relieve menopausal symptoms. Testosterone also fights breast cancer by increasing the activity and number of T cells that carry out cellular immunity. T killer cells kill cancer cells.

If you have estrogen-receptor-positive breast cancer and want to accept the risk of recurrence that might exist from estrogen replacement, nonoral estradiol is the safest estrogen in terms of avoiding breast cancer cell stimulation during replacement. The highest-risk replacement is oral estrogen because it turns into a large amount of estrone (the "old lady" estrogen, remember). Estrone can come from oral estrogen metabolism, from the adrenal gland, or belly fat and is more dangerous in terms of stimulating abnormal breast cells than estradiol. You should also be aware that taking estradiol through subdermal pellets avoids this concern because it does not convert into estrone in 90 percent of the women who take it.

As was mentioned earlier, the other exception to the rule is women who have had stage 1 breast cancer and had a bilateral mastectomy, with or without reconstruction. In this case, if there was no spread of cancer outside the breast and it is removed, estradiol may be replaced.

Until more research is done, oral estrogen should not be given to women with estrogen-receptor-positive breast cancer, other than the exceptional cases listed above. Other types of breast cancer are not affected by estrogen replacement.

New information and treatment strategies are being uncovered every day. Please discuss this with your physician for further information.

Personal History of Uterine Cancer

If you have had uterine cancer that extended beyond the uterus, estrogen is generally not given because it can stimulate dormant cells in the abdomen even after a hysterectomy. If the uterine cancer was limited to the uterine cavity and you had a hysterectomy, estrogen replacement is not considered high risk. If the cancer had spread to the lymph nodes, the only replacement therapy that should be provided is testosterone. Once again, testosterone does *not* stimulate any cancers in women.

Estrogen has specific risks that may or may not happen to you if you take estradiol. Side effects are dependent on how you genetically metabolize estrogen and other medications you take, as well as lifestyle choices. You may never have any of these problems, or you may have one or more of them; however, the good news is that most risks are not life threatening. Further detail on risks and side effects follows.

THE RISK AND SIDE EFFECTS OF ERT FOR WOMEN WHO HAVE NO CONTRAINDICATIONS

For women who do not have a medical history that prevents them from taking estradiol, there are still risks and possible side effects that are important to know before beginning ERT or HRT for the first time.

General Risks of ERT
Blood clots and pulmonary emboli (life threatening)
Breast cysts
Breast tenderness
Growth of uterine fibroids
Irregular and/or heavy bleeding
Postmenopausal bleeding: uterine
Uterine cancer (life threatening)
Water retention

Postmenopausal Bleeding: Uterine Bleeding

Postmenopausal bleeding is defined as any regular or irregular bleeding after you have missed 12 months of periods, or after you are technically in menopause. If this occurs after you take ERT or HRT, an ultrasound of the lining of the uterus is recommended to see if the bleeding is from a thick uterine lining, a very thin lining, a uterine polyp, a fibroid, or for no reason we can see—which means it is usually an imbalance between estrogen and progesterone. Bleeding is the most frequent side effect for women who have a uterus and take any type of estrogen.

When the uterus is exposed to estrogen, it wakes up, thickens its lining, and grows back to normal thickness, just like before menopause. Sometimes other dormant benign (noncancerous) growths such as polyps and uterine fibroids come to life, growing and bleeding as well. The risk of cancer of the endometrium (uterine lining) only becomes an issue after long-term (many years') exposure to estrogen without progesterone to balance it. This type of cancer is called endometrial cancer and is the most curable of all female cancers. Cancer of the uterus is not common because in the 1970s doctors began adding a progestin to all estrogen replacement, and the incidence of endometrial cancer in the U.S. and Canada became very low. Even though this is the only cancer that is increased in postmenopausal women who take HRT, it is the most treatable female cancer and is generally cured through a simple hysterectomy.

When postmenopausal bleeding is caused by a hormonal imbalance and not a physical abnormality that can be seen on ultrasound, the diagnosis is made by checking hormone levels and adding more progesterone.

Growth of Uterine Fibroids

Fibroids are benign, estrogen-sensitive muscle growths found in the uterus. They can cause postmenopausal bleeding and can grow under the influence of estrogen from any source, including ERT. In unusual cases ERT can make the fibroids grow or bleed, or both. A growing uterus might lead to a hysterectomy because of pain from pressure on other organs or intractable bleeding, so this risk should be considered when beginning ERT, especially if you have previously been told that you have fibroids.

Breast Tenderness and Breast Cysts

Estrogen (estradiol) stimulates normal breast tissue after the senescence (sleep from lack of estrogen) caused by menopause. Menopausal breasts look "deflated" in thin women and "over-stuffed" and droopy in overweight women. The best answer short of plastic surgery is estradiol replacement with testosterone. Breasts that are stimulated by estradiol and testosterone fill out and look perkier and younger. The side effect of this "reawakening" is that active breasts often grow cysts and become tender. This occurs most often during the first few months of estrogen replacement, and subsides thereafter. Tender and cystic breasts are not dangerous or a sign of breast cancer; however, ERT can make the breasts look denser on mammograms, which may make a mammogram more difficult to read accurately.

The most common cause of breast pain is not just estrogen (estradiol), but estrone. Another cause of breast tenderness is low iodine, common in Midwestern women, and low testosterone, which causes an increase in estrone. Try tolerating this side effect for a few months before abandoning ERT because it does not generally continue. Temporary therapy for breast tenderness and cysts includes 12.5 mg of Iodoral per day with a salty food, or you may choose to take DIM to decrease breast cysts and tenderness.

Whether you are on estradiol or not, any breast masses you find should be evaluated. Patients on estrogen replacement are at less risk for life-threatening breast cancer than if they had taken nothing at all after menopause. Anyone on or off estrogen replacement can get breast cancer, but it is not considered causative. Breast cancer takes between 7 to 12 years to grow from one abnormal cell to a mass large enough to be detected by any current radiologic technique. Women who believe their breast cancer was stimulated by estrogen replacement that was initiated less than seven years earlier are almost certainly incorrect. The growth pattern of breast cancers researched in many studies disproves this myth.

The replacement of estrogen can be extremely beneficial to women after menopause, and the benefits outweigh the risks. Recent research finds that women who have breast cancer diagnosed while they are on replacement estrogen have the most treatable cancers and a better survival rate than women who do not replace their estrogen after menopause.

Water Retention and Swelling

Water retention is a problem that most women deal with throughout their lives, long before ERT becomes necessary. The difference is that before menopause, water retention is cyclic and can be tolerated because of the promise of relief after a period. With ERT, unfortunately, it can be a daily issue. Sometimes diuretics and/or a high-protein, low-salt diet can solve the problem. Often the cause of swelling and water retention may be a reaction to the type of estrogen taken (most commonly synthetic, oral estrogen) or a thyroid malfunction in response to the added estradiol.

In short, the side effects of estrogen replacement are not severe in most women. They are easy to minimize by changing the type of estrogen or adding a supplement or medication to relieve these bothersome symptoms. The importance of choosing the estrogen that is most agreeable to your metabolism and troubleshooting any of these problems cannot be overemphasized. If estradiol is important to your feeling whole after menopause, it is worth the work to find the best kind of estrogen for your particular situation, with the fewest side effects.

Did you know that Oil of Olay contained estrogen back in the 1960s, and that was the key active ingredient that made it better than all other facial moisturizers? Estrogen after menopause is very good for skin, but it was removed from the cream out of fear of uterine cancer without testing the absorption from this effective face cream. In the case of estrogen replacement, we should review the most recent studies over the last ten years and acknowledge that the benefits greatly outweigh the risks when estrogen is given appropriately.

In recent years we have switched our fear from uterine cancer to breast cancer. We found a way to prevent uterine cancer while taking HRT, but the underlying distrust of estrogen replacement lives on in the threat of breast cancer. This fear is easier to refute now that many studies before and after the WHI study have proven it is safe, with some forms being safer than others. Breast cancer is much more likely to occur in obese women who don't exercise and who smoke than in those who take estrogen.

Uterine Cancer

Estrogen, whether supplied through replacement or naturally produced by the ovary, stimulates the growth of the uterine lining under normal circumstances. Progesterone decreases the growth of that same lining. After menopause, when ERT is taken without progesterone, the lining of the uterus grows without limits. The thicker the lining gets, the more abnormal the cells become. When the lining is greater than 4 to 5 mm after menopause, it should be evaluated for cancer. It is for this reason that doctors do not prescribe estrogen replacement without progesterone if the patient has a uterus.

Estrogen in nonoral bio-identical formulations prescribed with bio-identical progesterone is the key to successful treatment. Unless there is a polyp, fibroid, or excessive uterine lining before estrogen is replaced, estradiol and progesterone can be given safely without increasing the side effects of the treatment. The majority of women without a uterus do not need progesterone.

Estrogen Replacement Does Not Increase the Risk of Developing Breast Cancer

There are many risk factors that can increase your risk of getting breast cancer and some of these are avoidable, but the use of estrogen (without synthetic progestin) after menopause does not increase your risk of developing it. You can decrease your risk by changing your lifestyle. Of course, none of us can change our genetics or our medical or family history, but by achieving an ideal weight and refraining from bad habits we can hedge our bets and decrease our risk of getting breast cancer.

Factors That Increase the Risk of Developing Breast Cancer

- Abdominal Fat
- Current pregnancy
- Diabetes
- Excessive alcohol consumption
- Family history of breast cancer (mother, sister, aunt)
- Genetic defect called aromatization enzyme defect
- Having no children or having first child after age 30
- High amount of animal fat consumed
- Immune deficiency
- Italian, Sicilian, or Greek heritage
- Obesity
- Personal history of colon or ovarian cancer
- Race
- Radiation therapy to chest
- Sedentary lifestyle
- Smoking tobacco

The actual mechanism for the development of any cancer is the breakdown of the immune system—which happens with age, stress, or illness—and breast cancer is no exception. Everyone makes abnormal cells in every tissue of the body, every day. This fact is well documented and is part of being human. Because mistakes happen during the division of cells, they divide and give birth to cells that have critical abnormalities, which are sometimes cancer cells. The immune system is supposed to take care of us and kill cancer cells with T killer cells and other white blood cells that act as sentries for the body by seeking out and killing abnormal-appearing cells. When testosterone decreases with age, immune cells drop in number and activity and abnormal cells are not killed, so they multiply and grow into cancer. It is the strength of the immune system that combats these cancer cells and keeps us healthy. As women age, the hormones of their youth decline and so do the immune cells. In the context of aging, testosterone and growth hormone stimulate the activity and number of T cells when they are young. It is no wonder that replacement of testosterone is the most effective treatment for avoiding the occurrence of breast cancer.

Testosterone deficiency is the trigger for impaired immunity after 40 and places us in a position of vulnerability to cancer, so it is only logical that replacing that hormone would be the most efficient prevention. Testosterone also has a second way of stimulating the immune system; it competes with estradiol for receptor sites on breast cells and blocks the ability of estradiol and estrone to stimulate breast cells. In this way, testosterone modulates breast growth and diminishes the stimulation that estrogen might have on breast tissue.

We suggest a supplement that decreases estrone, which we mentioned earlier: DIM (diindolylmethane), a supplement made from cauliflower and broccoli. It works by blocking an enzyme reaction that converts testosterone into estrone. DIM decreases the amount of estrone in the body and in the breast, which decreases breast size, overall body fat, and breast cell turnover. This decreases the risk that a cell in the breast can become cancerous. This supplement is similar to Arimidex (an aromatase inhibitor), which is currently used to prevent and treat estrogen-receptor-positive breast cancer by decreasing estrone.

The results of medical studies investigating the role of ERT and breast cancer, after the WHI study, have been encouraging to those physicians and women who believe replacing estrogen after menopause is safe in regard to breast cancer. The majority of the subsequent studies revealed that the presence of progestin and the addition of testosterone are both factors that modify the risk of breast cancer. Progestin increases the risk of breast cancer while testosterone decreases the risk.

Follow-up studies of the WHI data revealed that the presence of an oral progestin plus estrogen did increase the rate of breast cancer above the risk for women who took nothing for menopause, but the lowest rate of breast cancer was for the women who took only estrogen replacement.

Testosterone was added to the mix in an Australian study by Dr. Constantine Dimitrakakis that was published in 2004 in the *Journal of Menopause*. In this artcle, Dr. Dimitrakakis provided data comparing the rates of breast cancer in women who never took hormone replacement; synthetic estrogen and progestin; estrogen, progestin, and testosterone; and testosterone alone. He found the choice of testosterone only to be the safest in regard to breast cancer. In all cases, adding testosterone decreased the number of patients who got breast cancer. The table on the next page summarizes the outcome of this study.

It is important to note that estrogen does not prevent breast cancer, but Leon Speroff, MD, the father of gynecological endocrinology, believes that if a woman who takes ERT gets breast cancer, she is more likely to survive compared to a woman who has never taken ERT!

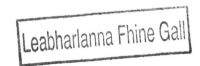

RISK OF BREAST CANCER PER 100,000 WOMAN YEARS*

HORMONE EXPOSURE	# OF WOMEN WITH BREAST CANCER
NEVER TOOK HORMONE REPLACEMENT	283
SYNTHETIC ESTROGEN + PROGESTIN	380
ESTROGEN + PROGESTIN + TESTOSTERONE	293
TESTOSTERONE ONLY	238

Dimitrakakis, et al. Menopause 11 (S): 531–535 September/October 2004

Women have a much greater chance of getting breast cancer if they do not use testosterone. The safest hormone replacement to avoid breast cancer is testosterone only replacement.

*Woman Years: the number of women in the study times the number of years they were studied equals 100,000.

Which Type of Estradiol Replacement Has the Best Benefit-Risk Ratio?

Estrogen has been prescribed by doctors as hormone replacement for menopause since the 1930s, and one of the first replacements was with bio-identical estradiol pellets placed under the skin. In following years, researchers began to look for other ways to formulate estrogen because in the 1930s and 1940s problems existed with the insertion process, and many of the pellets came out through the incision point. In addition, the pellets were not as advanced as they are now. As a result, physicians looked for a way to deliver oral estrogen without destroying it when it passed through the stomach. The original problem now rarely occurs, so the benefit of estradiol pellets outweighs the risks. Estradiol pellets now maintain the safest risk ratio among all ERT options.

Benefits of Progesterone Replacement

Progesterone replacement is one of the safest hormones women can take, although progesterone is not always necessary after menopause. Most women feel healthy and balanced when their estradiol and testosterone are replaced without progesterone. Only a very small percentage of women need progesterone to balance the other two hormones and treat their symptoms after menopause. In general, progesterone is given only to protect the uterus, not to treat symptoms after menopause.

The role of progesterone after childbearing is to protect the uterus from abnormal bleeding and uterine cancer. If you have a uterus and take estradiol replacement, you need to take progesterone to protect the uterus. If you have had a hysterectomy, progesterone is not prescribed. Prior to menopause, progesterone is necessary to balance the estradiol you produce in your ovary as you pass from the fertile stage of life to the premenopausal stage when estradiol levels are high and progesterone levels are low. Low progesterone levels prior to menopause and after age 40 cause abnormal periods, severe bleeding, growth of fibroids, and PMS. Replacing progesterone in the natural form, in a nonoral type of medication, relieves all of these symptoms.

Just to recap, progesterone aids in the following areas:

- Decreases menstrual cycle, menstrual flow
- Helps sleep and relieves anxiety
- Sometimes shrinks fibroids
- Treats PMS

These benefits are well known, and as long as progesterone is used in nonoral bio-identical form, the benefits are very obvious to the premenopausal patient who may have already gone through TDS.

Benefits for menopausal women are fewer. In general, the soothing capability of progesterone is very helpful in women who have anxiety problems after menopause. Progesterone replacement can also help women who have trouble falling asleep (not staying asleep) if it is dosed before bedtime. The primary reason for pre-scribing progesterone after menopause, however, is not treating symptoms but preventing uterine cancer when estrogens are given. Giving progesterone with estrogen replacement is why it is now safe to take estrogens. When women took estrogen in the 1950s and 1960s, this was not yet known and they took just estrogen for menopausal symptoms, even when they had a uterus.

RISKS OF PROGESTERONE REPLACEMENT

The risks of taking *progesterone* versus *progestin* are completely different, and we will only review the risks of *progesterone* replace-ment in depth because it is the only progesterone Kathy recom-mends. However, it is important to know the difference.

Side effects of nonoral progesterone replacement include mostly unpleasant symptoms, not life-threatening illness. The symptoms some women complain of are excessive hunger, fatigue, nausea, swelling, more bleeding instead of less, loss of hair, painful inter-course from a dry vagina, darkening of the facial skin in a masklike pattern, irritability, dry eyes, and a feeling of being unwell. For these reasons other methods to protect the uterus can be used to balance estradiol. These options include uterine ablation (surgical), Mirena IUD with a small bit of progestin on it to decrease bleeding, or observation yearly with an ultrasound to make sure the uterine lining doesn't get too thick.

Before menopause most women don't have symptoms from progesterone because it is a hormone their ovary produces at ovu-lation. Because bio-identical forms of this hormone are identical to what the body makes, they are the most effective and least risky for replacement. Progestins, on the other hand, are synthetic chemicals that look similar to progesterone but are processed differently in the body, and therefore have very different effects. Progestins (Aygestin, Provera, Depo-Provera) have been used for years in combination with oral estrogens, and they have been found to cause an increased occurrence of breast cancer. Bio-identical nonoral progesterone, however, has not been found to cause breast cancer.

There are no known medical risks for taking bio-identical progesterone. In terms of treatment of active breast cancer with positive progesterone markers, progesterone is avoided in any form, but there is no definitive research that proves that this improves breast cancer outcomes, and physiologically it doesn't make sense because progesterone decreases cell multiplication.

Who Can and Who Can't Take Progesterone

In general any woman can take progesterone if it is not given orally and is bio-identical. Some women have side effects from progesterone even if given as a pellet or sublingual (under the tongue) tablet. Progesterone is a natural relaxant; it makes some people sleepy or tired. For this reason, many women have trouble taking progesterone even if they need it to protect their uterus with ERT. Women who have PMS seem to need it, so they don't generally get the fatigue and sleepy side effects.

Most women find nonoral progesterone to be a diuretic, which reduces their water weight and swelling from estradiol replacement; however, some women find it causes swelling and water retention. These women have had the same reaction to birth control pills and often refuse progesterone. The last and most problematic side effect of progesterone is hunger. Most of us are opposed to any medication that causes weight gain, and this side effect is a very difficult one to conquer.

Countering the Side Effects of Progesterone

If progesterone is prescribed to treat a symptom like PMS or heavy menstrual bleeding, the treatment time is generally moderately short and some symptoms can be tolerated until the medical problem is resolved. On the other hand, if progesterone is given in combination with estradiol to prevent uterine bleeding and uterine cancer, the side effects will have to be endured or alternative methods of prevention must be employed.

Kathy's suggestion for those who cannot tolerate any kind of progesterone is to get an annual uterus ultrasound. If the lining is abnormal and thickened from estradiol replacement, they will have to undergo a biopsy of the lining of the uterus, or a D&C. Other women prefer very low doses of estradiol and will undergo biopsy if they have uterine bleeding during ERT.

Remember: progesterone is often given as a preventive hormone replacement and is very safe in terms of preventing uterine cancer and having a very low risk profile.

Hormone balance is key to good health and a long, productive life. Replacing all hormones whose deficiency causes aging and poor health is extremely important, but making sure hormonal balance is maintained on a 24-hour basis throughout each month and year is the goal of treatment. This generally requires limiting risks and maximizing benefits, as well as keeping every hormone balanced. This is not an easy mission but one an experienced doctor can walk you through. Our next chapter will utilize this information to help you develop a plan for your personal hormone replacement.

CHAPTER 9

How to Make the Best Choice in Hormone Replacement

How do you know whether you need to replace testosterone, progesterone, and/or estradiol? You may have symptoms of testosterone, progesterone, and estradiol deficiency, or your family history suggests that you are at risk for the diseases of long-term testosterone or estradiol deficiency, but how can you come to a decision? The process of deciding for yourself, along with your doctor's advice, must be logical and personal, and fit your lifestyle and medical history. After you have made your decision, testing will be necessary so your doctor can document your need for replacement therapy. In this chapter we will walk you through the steps that will end with a personal treatment plan for you.

We will use questionnaires to help you make a decision that fits your personal needs. Having read the information in the previous chapters, you may already have an idea about how hormone replacement could fit your needs. We will help you pull together the information you need so you can discuss this with your doctor.

First, it's important for you to know a little bit about the differences among synthetic, natural, and bio-identical hormones.

Synthetic hormones are chemicals made into a substance that acts similarly, but not identically, to the original hormone they are replacing. They do not chemically look like the body's hormone. In the lab, side chains are added to the original hormone to make it possible to take the pill orally; another chain is added to make it absorb slowly. (Remember this is the process of creating in the lab a "drug" that does not exist in nature but needs to mimic those that do exist in its operation so the body can metabolize it in the same way.) Natural hormones are destroyed in the stomach, so the producers of synthetic hormones alter their natural structure to make it possible to deliver them orally. The changes that are made in the lab cause side effects, so they are not the optimal replacement choice. In short, synthetic hormones are made from chemicals that are not found in the human body and are not identical in structure to human hormones.

Natural hormones are made from vegetables, not from a chemical base. Natural estradiol, testosterone, and progesterone are made from either yams or soy.

Bio-identical hormones describes the structure of replacement hormones. These are chemically identical in structure and function to the hormone secreted before menopause. Synthetic hormones are rarely identical and are made from chemicals other than plants. Therefore, bio-identicals have fewer side effects and better symptom relief than synthetic hormone replacement.

Now, let's start by finding out whether you qualify for hormone replacement.

Questionnaire #1: Are You a Candidate for Hormone Replacement?

Are you a candidate for testosterone replacement?

- ❑ Are you over 38, have completed childbearing, and have permanent birth control (UD, tubal ligation, or vasectomy of partner)?

- ❑ Are you menopausal, at any age?

❏ Have you had a hysterectomy and/or had your ovaries removed?

If you answered "yes" to any of these questions, you are a candidate for testosterone replacement.

Are you a candidate for progesterone replacement?

❏ Do you have symptoms of PMS during the two weeks before your period?

❏ Do you have a uterus and take estradiol replacement?

❏ Do you have trouble falling asleep during the last two weeks of your menstrual cycle, or after menopause?

❏ Do you have estrogen dominance and are cycling?

If you answered "yes" to any of these questions, you are a candidate for progesterone replacement.

Are you a candidate for estradiol replacement?

❏ Do you have symptoms of menopause: hot flashes, night sweats, dry vagina, and or no periods for more than 12 months?

❏ Do you have an FSH blood level over 23 MIUs twice in a month?

❏ Have you had your ovaries removed?

❏ Are you over 35 and have not had a period for a year?

❏ Do you have premature ovarian failure?

If you answered "yes" to any of these questions, you are a candidate for estradiol replacement.

Use the lines below to make note of the hormone(s) for which you are a candidate:

_____

_____

If you have determined that you are a candidate for replacement of at least one hormone, the next step is to uncover your true feelings about replacing your hormones. These questions are not as medically certain as those concerning hormone levels, but this questionnaire can help you find out if you are willing to accept treatment for your symptoms now, should choose to wait, or prefer to endure your symptoms instead of seeking treatment.

Questionnaire #2: How Do You Feel about Replacing Your Hormones?

The following statements are from real patients as they consider hormone replacement and indicate whether they are emotionally and physically prepared to replace their decreasing hormones. Please circle all of the letters that apply to you and then follow the directions that match your responses. For each of your answers, we have given guidance specifically designed to help you decide whether or not you are ready for hormone replacement.

A. I have enough symptoms of estrogen and testosterone deficiency that replacement might or certainly would improve my quality of life.

B. I have no symptoms of hormone deficiency, and my life is great as it is.

C. I am miserable, but I want to wait until something terrible happens before I make the decision to take hormones.

D. I am miserable and I cannot, or do not want to, continue my life as I know it without something to help me regain my health and quality of life.

E. I am already taking estrogen and/or testosterone in some form, but I want a more effective hormone replacement that will completely bring me back to health.

F. I just can't take another pill, or whatever! Leave me alone.

G. I will take herbs or vitamins, but no medicines, please.

H. I hate doctors, so forget it.

I. No matter how bad it is I will not change the course of nature. I don't want it!

A. You are possibly a good candidate for estrogen and testosterone replacement, so now let's look at the risks and benefits and decide if you have any risks that might prevent your use of either hormone.

B. You are a lucky woman! You have great genetics and have led a healthy life, or you have not progressed far enough into menopause or TDS to be symptomatic. Thank your lucky stars and God, and keep your eye out for any deficiency symptoms.

C. You are a woman who waits for a crisis to manage your health problems. If this is really how you would like to proceed, please revisit this test when one of the diseases of TDS or menopause occurs and begin the tests again.

D. You are in need of hormone replacement! Please proceed to the risks section and view the possible downside to therapy. If your current situation is more risky or miserable than the risks, we can help you through the risks in several ways.

E. You are a good candidate for hormone replacement! Even though you probably know the risks of hormone therapy, check with your doctor.

F. You are sick and obviously too stressed to consider a change, even one for the better. Please pick up this book again when you are not so overwrought because you of all women who read it could benefit the most!

G. We understand that you prefer natural treatments over prescriptions, but remember that we are discussing bio-identical hormones that are made from vegetables, not chemicals. If it is control of the replacement you are concerned about, you may do best with a vaginal tablet or transdermal replacement.

H. If you hate doctors, we understand, but you should not allow your fear or anger to keep you from the fullest, healthiest life possible. Give hormone replacement and yourself a chance to help you get healthy.

I. We know lots of women like you! You are concerned with mucking around with the natural course of things, so you are willing to sacrifice your health, sex life, and energy to keep the status quo. If so, hang on to this book because when aging deals you the cards of pain, disease, and loss of the youthful ability to get around easily, you might reconsider. For now, I wish you the best!

If you have made it this far and are a candidate for or want hormone replacement, hang in there. You will begin to see the advantage of replacing the hormones that disappear with age!

As we know from the last chapter, it is important to review the risks of replacing your hormones individually. The next questionnaire will determine whether you are at high risk for complications, side effects, or new symptoms, broken out by each hormone's specific risks. Once you know the risks, you can decide whether to take those risks or not. Some risks have treatments that make them safe, and they will be discussed as well.

Questionnaire #3: What Are Your Risks with Testosterone Replacement?

Please circle all of the letters that apply to you and then follow the directions that match your responses.

A. I have a history of a liver tumor. I have been told not to take oral hormones of any kind.

B. I do not want facial hair under any circumstances.

C. My voice is important to me because I am a singer, and/or I need it to sound the same at all times, and testosterone could lower my voice.

D. It is important to me that I do not gain muscle mass.

E. I do not want acne or oily skin.

F. I am not interested in increasing my desire for sex.

G. My hair is thin and I do not want to take testosterone because I hear that it will make my hair fall out.

H. I am afraid of clitoral enlargement even though I know it has gotten smaller since my testosterone has decreased.

I. I am afraid of testosterone because I hear it will make me into a man.

J. I have an autoimmune disease such as lupus, MS, scleroderma, or rheumatoid arthritis.

K. I have had breast cancer and was told I cannot take hormones.

L. I have no risk factors.

A. *You may take any type of testosterone replacement except oral testosterone. You are not at risk of any growth or medical complications from testosterone replacement.*

B. *Facial hair is increased with testosterone replacement of any kind, but it is easily prevented with one of two drugs, spironolactone tablets or finasteride. If you don't want to take a medication, then waxing, laser, epilation, or bleaching are adequate treatments. Testosterone is so effective and beneficial that you should not refuse treatment for such a minor cosmetic problem.*

C. *Women's voices are higher in pitch because men have a normal free testosterone level ten times higher than normal free testosterone levels of women. The effect on the voice is entirely dose dependent on testosterone as well as balanced by estradiol levels. Be sure to tell your physician to minimize the dose of testosterone to protect your voice.*

D. *Healthy muscle mass is just that: good for you! Your muscles are meant to burn calories and support your frame, including your joints and your back. Without muscles you will look thinner, but you are not leaner without muscles. This is one of those healthy benefits of testosterone, so you should embrace it!*

E. *Acne and oily skin are truly a side effect of testosterone on the skin. If you had oily skin as a young person you may get it again from the replacement of testosterone. The same medications that prevent facial hair (spironolactone tablets and finasteride) also block the effects of testosterone on the oil glands of the skin.*

F. *Not desiring a libido is reasonable, especially if you do not have a partner, but a sex drive is a normal facet of the human personality and has many acceptable outlets other than sexual activity. Some women solve the problem with a vibrator or by reading erotic literature. Having a sex drive does not mean you will act on the desire.*

G. *Thin hair after 40 can be caused by various changes: frontal hair loss is usually due to loss of estradiol, and loss at the temples and crown is secondary to a metabolite of testosterone, DHT. Hair thinning over the whole head is often due to low thyroid hormone. If this occurs with your replacement, the medications finasteride and/or spironolactone can be used to thicken low testosterone–induced hair loss.*

H. Clitoral enlargement is not harmful, even though some doctors may act like it is a disease. The clitoris generally decreases in size as the body becomes accustomed to the hormone levels.

I. Testosterone won't make you turn into a man. Men have ten times as much free testosterone as women have and they have different receptor sites. Female receptor sites share their activity with estradiol, so our response is quite different from men's. Don't worry: becoming less feminine by replacing testosterone is an old wives' tale.

J. Autoimmune diseases are improved by the presence of testosterone. We treat patients with these illnesses with testosterone pellets, and they improve greatly. Estradiol can have a negative effect on autoimmune diseases, but testosterone can balance out the effect and allow women to take both testosterone and estradiol.

K. Breast cancer is not caused by testosterone; in fact, testosterone prevents the development of all cancers by stimulating the immune system.

L. If you have no reason to avoid testosterone, talk to your doctor about your options.

Now we will evaluate your risks for progesterone replacement. Progesterone is very low in risk but some women cannot take progesterone for various reasons. If you are premenopausal, then proceed with the questionnaire. If you are postmenopausal and have had a hysterectomy or your ovaries have been removed, or you have a Mirena IUD or ablation, you do not need progesterone. Skip this questionnaire and move on to the risks of estradiol questionnaire.

Questionnaire #4: What Are Your Risks with Progesterone Replacement?

Please circle all of the letters that apply to you and then follow the directions that match your responses.

A. When I take progesterone, I bleed instead of stopping bleeding as I expected to.

B. When I take progesterone, I feel nauseated, irritable, and/or swollen.

C. When I take progesterone, I have fatigue and gain weight immediately.

D. Progesterone gives me a dry vagina and dry eyes.

A. Some women have an opposite response to progesterone and cannot take it in any form. It is important to stop trying other forms of progesterone if bleeding is a response to progesterone; it won't work. Instead of progesterone, you can try taking birth control pills or use a Mirena IUD.

B. If you have these side effects in response to progesterone, it is probably not safe for you to take it. You should find another way to protect your uterus after menopause. You may want to have a surgical ablation or use a Mirena IUD. If you have PMS and cannot take progesterone, you should try a low-dose antidepressant to treat your symptoms.

C. Weight gain from progesterone is highest in any oral form and lowest in transdermal form. When it is accompanied by fatigue, taking it at night is much more palatable, and decreasing the dose is also helpful to accommodate and avoid the side effects.

D. If you have one or both of these side effects, bio-identical progesterone is less likely to cause these problems, and the addition of estradiol and testosterone generally overcome this irritating side effect.

Progesterone, as we have said before, is generally needed for PMS before menopause and only to balance the effect of estradiol on the lining of the uterus so women can take estradiol safely.

Estradiol is the third and final hormone needed to counteract the symptoms of aging. It is the last to disappear and the most common hormone to be replaced. This hormone also has some of the most discussed risks, some of which are not real. Please take the next questionnaire to see what risks might occur if you replace estradiol and how to ameliorate them so replacing estradiol remains possible.

Questionnaire #5: What Are Your Risks with Estradiol Replacement?

Please circle all of the letters that apply to you and then follow the directions that match your responses.

A. I have had a DVT (deep venous thrombosis) or a PE (pulmonary embolism) (not including clotted varicose veins or IV sites).

B. I have a family history of breast cancer (two or more—either a sister, mother, or aunt).

C. I have had invasive breast cancer with estrogen receptors.

D. I have had invasive breast cancer without estrogen receptors.

E. I have had breast cancer with positive estrogen receptors that was stage 1 or less, I had no positive nodes, and I have had a bilateral mastectomy.

F. I could not take birth control pills because of side effects.

G. I have or had uterine cancer that spread outside of the uterus.

H. I have no high-risk problems, but I can't take progesterone to balance estradiol.

I. I have an autoimmune disease such as lupus, MS, scleroderma, or rheumatoid arthritis.

J. I have had a hysterectomy.

K. I smoke cigarettes.

L. I have no risk factors.

A. You may or may not be able to take estrogen without the risk of another blood clot or pulmonary embolism; it all depends on your genetics. The various genetic tests required to determine whether you are at risk for another event are discussed in Chapter 8. If your blood test is negative for genetic risk factors, you are at no more risk than anyone else of getting a DVT or embolism.

B. Your family history puts you at a 50 percent risk of getting breast cancer during your lifetime, with or without estrogen replacement. You can still take estrogen if you decrease your risk by taking nonoral estradiol, adding nonoral testosterone, and taking either DIM (a nutritional supplement that decreases estrone) or Arimidex (aromatase enzyme inhibitor) to protect you from the cancer.

C. Invasive breast cancer with estrogen receptors makes taking estrogen in any form risky. Our advice is to take nonoral testosterone and Arimidex, which together will decrease your risk of recurrence drastically—even lower than women who take nothing—and will improve your symptoms of TDS and menopause. Some women also add vaginal estrogen to locally relieve the dryness of menopause without influencing the cancer cells.

D. Invasive breast cancer without estrogen receptors is not affected by estradiol in a negative way. We have recently found that those patients who had been taking estrogen when their non–estradiol-receptor-positive cancers were found have less aggressive tumors.

E. Women who have had invasive breast cancer with estrogen receptors and a curative bilateral mastectomy are cleared by their oncologists to take estradiol. We suggest the nonoral, bio-identical type at a moderate dose to relieve symptoms of menopause. The addition of nonoral testosterone will improve immune function and decrease the risk of recurrence even more.

F. Side effects of birth control pills (BCPs) are a warning sign that you might get the same side effects from estrogen replacement, but only in the oral form or those with oral progestins. You can still take postmenopausal estradiol. The most common side effects from BCPs include decreased libido, nausea, vomiting, depression, and migraine headaches. The best method is to take your estradiol in a nonoral, bio-identical form with the least amount of nonoral progesterone possible. Choosing this type of estrogen and delivery system will make the appearance of the same side effects unlikely.

G. Uterine cancer that has been treated with a hysterectomy is generally completely resolved and does not place you at risk for recurrence from estrogens taken for menopause. If the spread was beyond the uterus, the usual treatment is nonoral testosterone. Discuss the treatment with your oncologist before proceeding with estrogen.

H. You are certainly able to take estrogen, but instead of progesterone, you must have another method of protecting your uterine lining from bleeding and cancer. The options are to have a Mirena IUD inserted, undergo an ablation of the lining of the uterus, have a hysterectomy, or monitor the uterine lining on a yearly basis with an ultrasound, and possibly an office endometrial biopsy to make sure there is no sign of uterine cancer.

I. Autoimmune diseases get worse when treated with estrogen alone, especially oral estrogen (with or without progestins). We do give estrogen to our patients with these diseases, but we keep the dose very low and always use a large dose of testosterone, because testosterone makes autoimmune diseases better.

J. Those with hysterectomies and no other risk factors may proceed to the types of estradiol and testosterone that are recommended. You should ask your doctor about a nonoral delivery system (such as a patch) with estrogen alone (meaning without progestin added).

K. Smoking cigarettes is a threat to your life—for breast cancer, lung cancer, and emphysema—but is not a risk for estrogen replacement.

L. No risk factors? Good for you! You can take estrogen.

Now that you've decided whether you are a candidate for hormone replacement; what your true feelings are regarding hormone replacement; and whether you are at high risk for any of the three hormones necessary to balance your hormonal environment, the next step is to review the lab values that confirm your need for each of the hormones of the aging cascade. You can refer to the blood testing section in Chapter 5. The presence of symptoms and qualifying blood levels for each hormonal deficit confirms the diagnosis.

Now we will look at how you can choose your type of hormone replacement.

Questionnaire #6: Which Results and Issues Matter to You in Your Testosterone Replacement?

The information in the following questionnaire is helpful in making a decision about the type of testosterone replacement that suits your needs.

Here you will rank the issues of various forms of testosterone replacement from most important to least important. Place a "1" next to the issue that is of most importance to you; "2" is second most important, and so on.

____   A.   I want the treatment that is most effective and will relieve all or almost all of my TDS symptoms.

____   B.   I want the treatment that is easiest to use and takes the least effort to dose.

____   C.   I want the treatment with the fewest side effects.

____   D.   I want the treatment that is covered by my insurance.

____   E.   I want the treatment that costs least.

If you chose A, pellets are most effective.

If you chose B, pellets are easiest to use.

If you chose C, pellets have the fewest side effects.

If you chose D, oral Estratest is your only covered option.

If you chose E, pellets are the least expensive.

Are Pellets Too Expensive to Consider?

As we discussed in Chapter 8, the average woman is spending about $251.50 a month in co-pays for a variety of medicines that she might be able to stop if she takes hormone pellets. The savings will cut her costs for medications almost in half if she takes testosterone and estrogen replacement with bio-identical pellets—her cost will drop to about $1,679 a year. This means her daily costs will drop from around $8.27 to about $4.60, saving almost four dollars a day in costs. So the point here is that you can save almost half of what you spend now and feel better for all the days you have.

Different Forms of Bio-identical Testosterone				
Delivery System of Testosterone	Use	Cost	Effectiveness	Negatives
Oral bio-identical	Once-daily pill	Bio-identical may not be covered by insurance	Moderate	• Converts into estrone • Mood issues with anger • Not effective for all symptoms of TDS
Sublingual bio-identical	One to two times daily	Not covered by insurance; about $100 a month	Minimal	Absorption rate poor
Vaginal	Once daily	Not covered by insurance; about $100 a month	Good	Fluctuation of levels in bloodstream causes relief to be intermittent
Creams (transdermal)	Apply every 4–6 hours	Not covered by insurance; about $100 a month	Minimal	Multiple applications a day; minimal response
Subdermal pellets	Inserted once every 4–6 months	$400–500 every 4–6 months	Excellent	Side effects of procedure

Clearly, testosterone pellets are an ideal choice for many women! Let's look more closely at what they are and why they're such an effective option.

What Exactly Is Hormone Pellet Therapy?

Hormone pellet therapy is a comprehensive look at blood work, a consultation that includes taking a medical history and a modified physical exam, postinsertion follow-up lab tests (with yearly follow-up labs), supplements to improve outcomes, diet to improve outcomes, treatment of other illnesses, and, as needed, consultation with other doctors.

Bio-identical hormone pellets are compounded (made and shaped) from the natural ingredients found in soy and yams. The varieties include estradiol, testosterone, and progesterone. They are chemically identical to the hormones produced in our ovaries until menopause and concentrated into pellets that can be inserted into the fat under the skin of the hip. In that site, the pellets dissolve slowly and completely. Pellets are BNDD controlled but not yet approved for female hormone replacement. No bio-identical hormones are approved by the FDA for use by women.

Pellets come from one of a multitude of compounding pharmacies scattered throughout the U.S. and Canada. The manufacture, distribution, and prescription use of pellets are controlled by FDA regulations, but the pellets are not approved for use in women, as we talked about in Chapter 2.

When considering hormone replacement, your doctor must make a decision about whether to replace estrogen, testosterone, and/or progesterone. Women make these three hormones during their youth. Every woman may need one, two, or all three to replace what is missing and to feel normal. The contraindications differ for each hormone and each woman, based on her history. Keep in mind that even if you can't take one of the three, it does not rule out the other two.

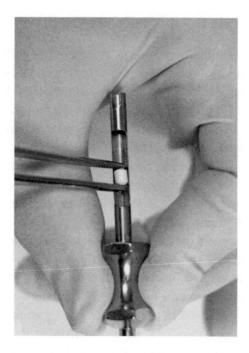

There are a few risks associated with pellet insertion:

- Allergy to lidocaine or epinephrine
- Allergy to the pellet itself or to medical tape
- Bruising and bleeding
- Granuloma, a reaction to infection or foreign body that causes a round mass form around the area of infection or the foreign body. It feels like a small, hard, round mass under the skin.
- Infection
- Keloids, a type of scar that is irregular and is raised above the skin. They are made of collagen, and progressively enlarge. They occur in genetically susceptible people.
- Pellet expulsion
- Scarring (minor)

There are steps you can take to minimize risks; for example, to decrease risk of bruising, stop all aspirin products three to seven days before insertion. Let your doctor know about any recent injuries in the area of the insertion. Notify him or her at the time of the procedure of any tendency to develop keloids, new medication, or medical diagnoses.

Testosterone Pellets Are the Superheroes of Testosterone Replacement

This is very nonscientific claim, but because Kathy was a patient who got her life back from testosterone pellet replacement and she's a doctor who has witnessed thousands of patients regain their health and happiness, it is her most truthful and powerful statement. We realize that advertisers say the same type of thing about everything from shampoo to herbal baths and supplements, but that does not make this statement less accurate. Here are some facts to support the legitimacy of this claim:

- Testosterone can only be replaced in a nonoral way to truly replicate the same action it had in the female body prior to age 40.

- Subdermal, time-release pellets are physiologically similar to how the ovary delivers testosterone, and that guarantees stable blood levels for months at a time.

- Testosterone delivered by pellets is the best form to adequately prevent breast cancer, Alzheimer's disease, other forms of dementia, heart disease, osteoporosis, sarcopenia, obesity, and other diseases of aging, because it creates the least amount of estrone.

- Pellet delivery *guarantees* delivery of the pure hormone every minute of every day, without effort on the part of the patient.

There are many other reasons we advocate for testosterone pellets, having to do with the failings of the other forms of, and delivery systems for, testosterone, and we have fully addressed these earlier in the book.

When patients come to us after seeing other doctors who use bio-identical estrogens plus or minus testosterone, we see the extraordinary difference in them after only one treatment with testosterone pellets. The difference is so dramatic that the before-and-after pictures we take are obvious to people on the street, who know nothing of the treatment that was used to turn these women back into their younger selves. Their faces glow while they exult about their recovery and their newly restored sexuality and health!

Sadly, pellet therapy is not yet universal, even though it is growing quickly in the U.S. There are not enough doctors properly trained and educated to accommodate all the women over 40. Until better information and education bring more doctors and more women to the realization that bio-identical pellets are the most successful treatment strategy, incorporating the least number of negatives for women over 40, we support the use of other types of bio-identical testosterone. In the current environment, we believe that some testosterone is better than none.

One of the major goals of this book is to spread the word to women that they need to generate an outcry for comprehensive replacement of testosterone for women. When we are able to receive testosterone as easily aging men do, our equality will be more complete.

Conversations with Physicians

Many of Kathy's colleagues ask, "Why do you use an expensive treatment like pellets when any bio-identical hormone replacement does the same thing?"

Here's what she tells them. Pellet testosterone and estradiol replacement are not the same as other forms of bio-identical hormones. The other forms may work a little with some patients, but testosterone pellets are 95 percent effective in the women she screens, and they resolve 100 percent of the symptoms attributable to testosterone deficiency.

Nonpellet hormone therapy may not work at all for her colleagues' patients for the following reasons:

1. Blood levels reveal that most patients do not absorb other nonoral forms of bio-identical hormones, or they are converted to 60 to 80 percent estrone ("old lady" estrogen).

2. FSH is not suppressed back to premenopausal levels by nonpellet forms of testosterone, so subtle surges of FSH/LH cause sleep disturbances, anxiety, and irritability, even with bio-identical replacement of other types.

3. Some bio-identical hormones are absorbed through the skin, through the vagina, or under the tongue and do not have the same effect. If you have tried one of these bio-identical delivery systems and were disappointed, *it does not mean* hormone pellets won't be the answer for you.

4. Only pellet bio-identical testosterone reestablishes the estradiol-estrone youthful ratio of 2:1, which is healthy and reverses aging.

This ratio is pivotal to feeling young and "normal" again. Women have a 2:1 ratio of young to "old lady" estrogen before menopause, and the only hormone replacement that brings women back to this normal ratio is pellets. All other forms have the opposite ratio, making women feel old and muddled.

Other doctors might ask about the expertise involved in pellet therapy. The truth is that pellet therapy with bio-identical estradiol and testosterone is both an art and a science. This practice requires an extensive knowledge of bio-identical hormones of all types, as well as training in the dosage and goals of hormone replacement therapy. In addition, doctors who provide hormone replacement therapies must be knowledgeable concerning *all* related hormone imbalances, such as hyperprolactinemia, hypo- and hyperthyroidism, pituitary tumors, brain injury hormone loss, adrenal fatigue, and Cushing's disease, as well as knowing how to treat growth hormone abnormalities.

The technique of inserting the pellets is a skill that requires adherence to sterile procedures and surgical training taught under the direct supervision of an established surgeon/physician. This is why I believe the best overlapping specialties for providing these treatments are OB/GYNs and family practitioners, because they have cross-training in surgery and knowledge of hormone systems.

Kathy always tells them that a gifted brain surgeon makes his surgeries look effortless, but they most certainly are not!

Choose Your Doctor Wisely!

We have heard many sad stories from patients about doctors attempting to provide these treatments without adequate training, resulting in traumatic insertions without proper incisions, and over- and underdosing, which set their bodies off on a roller coaster of hormone imbalances. It's important to standardize the methodology and make sure physicians are properly trained to treat their patients effectively.

When you ask your doctor about how they do pellets, ask them how many years they have done this and verify how they were trained. Doctors who really know how to diagnose and implement this therapy currently make up a very short list. You deserve the best treatment when it comes to your health.

Now that you have had an opportunity to examine the risks and benefits, your next step will be to speak with your physician and your partner to determine the best path forward, with full information and knowledge about your options. If your doctor is not familiar with this information, be sure to make them aware of the contents of this book. Remember that being an informed consumer of medical options is your right and your responsibility.

CONCLUSION

We came to write this book because we were increasingly frustrated by stories of women in midlife whose complaints had been ignored by the medical community. But this frustration gave us a rare and unexpected opportunity to blaze a trail on behalf of women everywhere.

In this book, our mission has been to educate women so that they are aware of *all* of their options. Our approach has been to walk through the natural progressive loss of hormones: the aging cascade that eventually leads all of us to old age. If upon reading this book, you feel that you or someone you love may be suffering from TDS, let this be a resource to help you identify your symptoms, consider your options, and select the path that works best for you. We encourage you to meet with your physician to discuss what you have learned, and bring along the questionnaires and data you've collected.

We hope this book sparks a revolution in the way the illnesses of aging among women are identified and treated. Over the years, we've experienced women, some of whom you have read about in this book, who have obtained *complete* symptom relief. They have joined the revolution. We hope that we've inspired you to join as well.

The tides of medicine change slowly and with great resistance, but they are changing. Right now, we are at the crest of a wave in women's health that will move the tide of medicine forward toward more knowledge and greater capacity to make preventive hormone replacement the standard of care.

CONCLUSION

APPENDIX A

Troubleshooting Hormone Replacement Therapy

The compilation of the long-term effects of hormonal deficiencies has been addressed in the medical text *The Hormone Handbook*, second edition, by Thierry Hertoghe, MD, a third-generation endocrinologist. We have updated the following table with the newest research, so it varies slightly from his findings. However, this is an excellent way to look up what you are at risk for if you don't replace the hormones that disappear with age.

Diseases Caused by Specific Hormone Deficiencies (Lack of Hormone)								
Hormone Deficiency	Heart Disease	High Blood Pressure	Breast Cancer	Diabetes	Osteoporosis	Anxiety/ Depression	Obesity	Dementia, Alzheimer's
Testosterone	Y	?	Y	Y	Y	Y	Y	Y
Estradiol	Y	Y	N	Y	Y	Y	Y	Y
Progesterone	?	?	?	?	Y	Y Anxiety	?	N
Thyroid	Y	Y	N	Y	N	Y	Y	Y
Cortisol	N	N	N	N	N	Y	N	N
Growth Hormone	Y	Y	N	Y	Y	Y	Y	Y

It is important to note that there are other hormones involved in antiaging that, when deficient, are also involved in susceptibility to the diseases of aging. When the hormones in the chart are present, they prevent the diseases listed in the chart.

A visual example can be made from the game of volleyball. When a ball comes over the net, the first person to hit the ball is the primary hormone (one of those listed in the chart), setting the ball up for another team member (stimulating other glands) to then hit the ball over the net, or make secondary hormones that also prevent the diseases mentioned.

The secondary hormones that are stimulated by the actions of testosterone are listed in the following chart. They produce a secondary system that prevents disease.

Hormones Testosterone Stimulates	Effects of Each Hormone
Calcitonin	Improves bone development
DHT	Builds muscle; improves strength; improves skin tone and moisture
Growth Hormone	Increases lean body mass and fat loss; increases energy, muscle growth, and bone development; improves skin tone, joint health, and support structures for bladder and skin
Melatonin	Induces sleep; increases weight loss; improves skin thickness and color; enhances the immune system; acts as an anti-inflammatory
Oxytocin	Improves orgasms and libido; calms mood; increases vaginal wetness, strength of orgasms, and vaginal ejaculation; stimulates breast tone
Thyroid	Increases metabolism; increases energy and growth of hair, nails, and bone; improves bowel health

For example, testosterone (by either replacement or natural production) stimulates the production of growth hormone, thyroid hormones, cortisol, and insulin.

We turn our focus to testosterone in this book for women because its presence both prevents many diseases on its own and stimulates the most beneficial antiaging hormones! It is by far the most efficient hormone to replace because it generally triggers the secretion of other beneficial hormones, balancing the system in fewer steps with fewer drugs (hormone replacements).

TESTOSTERONE REPLACEMENT: TROUBLESHOOTING

Testosterone is the most important and most efficient hormone to replace when dealing with the symptoms of aging and the symptoms of testosterone deficiency. In general, replacement of testosterone is extremely effective in most women and solves a multitude of problems in women over 40. In the case of side effects or poor response, there are several troubleshooting techniques that can make all the difference.

Several factors can interfere with the resolution of TDS symptoms in the area of energy and libido. The symptoms may not resolve in a woman when replaced with enough testosterone to achieve excellent blood levels of testosterone if a woman is taking multiple antidepressants, antianxiety medications, or drugs to treat manic-depressive disorder. These medications can counteract testosterone's benefits. The answer is to try to wean off these medications as mood improves on testosterone, under the direction of the doctor who provides care for the emotional issues.

When estradiol is very high (over 200), renewed testosterone levels may not renew sexuality and energy because testosterone competes for the receptor sites it shares with estradiol. Testosterone is not as good at binding to the receptors, so the high estradiol level impairs improvement of low-testosterone symptoms.

Why do some forms of testosterone—such as transdermal, oral, and sublingual—improve symptoms initially but stop working in a month or two?

These forms begin by delivering testosterone with a small amount of estrone that forms from testosterone's conversion as it goes through the skin, mucosa of the mouth, or vagina. With time, estrone increases and inactivates testosterone by making free testosterone (the active form) into bound testosterone. This progressively decreases the active form of testosterone, making the symptoms of low testosterone return.

Pellets and vaginal tablets do not convert into estrone except in women who have an aromatase enzyme defect secondary to their genetics.

Why is the Wylie Protocol ineffective for the symptoms of testosterone?

There is no testosterone in the Wylie program of multiple daily dosages of vaginal creams!

Does testosterone replacement help weight loss?

Women over 40 usually note that testosterone replacement doesn't always make them lose weight in the first four to six months, even with excellent dieting and exercise. But their waistlines do decrease when the right testosterone is administered and estrone is followed and controlled.

In general, testosterone is an anabolic hormone, meaning it builds muscle and bone when it reaches the right level. By replacing testosterone, bones and muscles regain their under-40 size and density, and thus weigh more than small muscles and thin bones. However, at the same time, testosterone decreases body fat, especially belly fat. For the first six months, the exchange of fat to muscle and bone keeps weight the same as the body's "volume" or size decreases. As muscle grows it burns calories all the time, and then weight decreases until ideal weight is reached.

If the side effect of testosterone is facial hair growth, what can be done about it?

Testosterone causes hair growth on some women's faces to a greater degree than it does on others. The degree of this problem depends on the density of receptors for the testosterone metabolite DHT (dihydrotestosterone). This means that the blood level of DHT doesn't always determine the level of facial hair, but genetics do!

Some troubleshooting for this problem comes in the form of several medications or supplements. We generally try saw palmetto, a supplement that is very effective in preventing facial hair. If the problem is more severe, the diuretic spironolactone or the medication finasteride (Propecia, Proscar) are both effective in preventing facial hair growth.

Of course, the aesthetic management of facial hair is always an option. This includes waxing, lasering, threading, epilation, and bleaching dark facial hair. Shaving is not an option because it leaves stubble.

Fatigue is sometimes not completely treated when testosterone has been prescribed.

Fatigue can be secondary to many imbalances, so all the other hormones that can be inadequate and cause fatigue should be evaluated and replaced if necessary. These hormones include thyroid hormone, cortisol, estradiol, adrenaline, norepinephrine, and dopamine.

Autoimmune diseases, chronic fatigue, chronic pain, and sleep apnea can also cause fatigue, hypothyroidism, and low cortisol, even if you are on testosterone.

Blood levels of free testosterone are not sufficient, and symptoms are not relieved.

Delivery of testosterone to the bloodstream is the most basic requirement leading to resolution of symptoms. The second and third issues are dosage and compliance: the amount of testosterone given and the frequency with which you actually take the testosterone at the right time. The type of testosterone is also a variable in the goal to achieve ideal blood levels of free testosterone.

ESTRADIOL REPLACEMENT: TROUBLESHOOTING

Estradiol is the second most important hormone to replace, but as with any medication or hormone replacement, it has some side effects that require your doctor's intervention.

Initial side effects of estrogen treatment: swelling

Fluid retention is the most common side effect of estrogen replacement. The oral preparations have the highest rate of swelling, so if you experienced this side effect in the past with birth control pills, either choose another way to take estrogen that rarely causes swelling and fluid retention (such as patches or pellets) or ask for a diuretic with your ERT to counteract this symptom. Adding natural progesterone in a nonoral delivery system like sublingual or pellet can help with swelling in some women, but this is not universal.

Celery; high-protein, low-carb shakes; and watermelon all decrease swelling. Did you know that for every gram of carbohydrate you eat in a day, you will gain a cc or milliliter of water? This supports the finding that high-protein shakes cause diuresis (urination) both because they increase the viscosity of the blood and because they decrease the possibility of high carbohydrate intake.

Estrogen replacement side effect: uterine bleeding

Any type of estrogen replacement may cause uterine bleeding, and the only surefire way to prevent that is a hysterectomy. If you are attached to your uterus, then the best way to avoid bleeding all together is to:

1. Get a Mirena IUD that stops bleeding for five years.
2. Have a uterine ablation to remove the tissue that bleeds monthly. This is about 85 percent effective.
3. Take constant progesterone by sublingual tablet, pellet, or vaginal tablet. Transdermal creams cause breakthrough bleeding and can allow buildup of the lining of the uterus, putting you at risk for uterine cancer.

Other women just want to continue periods, cleaning the uterus out each month, so for them, cyclic progesterone should be given for a week every month, and that will be followed by a period.

Breakthrough bleeding and/or heavy bleeding postmenopause

We troubleshoot this problem by first waiting it out if it occurs right after initiation of HRT. Then we double the amount of progesterone taken to balance the estrogen that is replaced. We generally follow this sequence:

1. Double progesterone dose.
2. Decrease estradiol dose.
3. Encourage weight loss.
4. Check hormone levels to see if estrone is high. Then give DIM supplement or Arimidex to stop estrone production that causes bleeding. Use ultrasound to find polyp, thickened lining, or fibroid growth. Perform an endometrial biopsy to rule out endometrial cancer (office procedure).

5. Perform a D&C or clean out the uterus to start at square one. (Make sure to ask for an ablation at the same time, so you don't have to keep doing that every year!)

Irritability and worsened anxiety with estrogen replacement of any type

Estradiol usually calms and ameliorates anxiety attacks caused by FSH surges (experienced as hot flashes), but there are some women who are "progesterone gals." If they take estrogen of any type, they feel anxious, as if they have never-ending PMS. These women truly require progesterone, in a natural form and nonorally, to keep them calm and allow them to sleep well. Progesterone gals are diagnosed without a test but with the medical instinct and observation of their doctor that comes with treating many women with hormones and asking the right questions.

When estradiol and progesterone don't assist women in getting sound sleep

After estradiol and progesterone are replaced, hot flashes and night sweats should cease and allow the woman to sleep soundly. Yet many patients don't have that benefit if only these two hormones are replaced. This can be for several reasons, the most common being a lack of testosterone. When testosterone is not replaced or is replaced in an oral form, sleep does not improve because the women who experience this issue can't enter stage 3 or 4 sleep and receive the healing and resting benefits of deep sleep without testosterone. Generally, 95 percent of patients sleep well if we just replace testosterone.

The other causes of poor quality sleep can include the following:

1. Cortisol production is elevated or is not normal with the diurnal pattern necessary for sleep.

2. Untreated ADD, sleep apnea, or narcolepsy cause the sympathetic nervous system to continue to fire all night, preventing restful sleep, and can cause restless leg syndrome. The treatments for these conditions lie in the purview of neurologists and psychiatrists, but typically include an amphetamine-like medication taken during the day that lasts about 12 hours so the nervous system will calm down at night.

3. Low melatonin can be the cause of ongoing sleep problems.

Overheating after ERT, HRT, and testosterone replacement

Body temperature is under the control of the hormones testosterone, thyroid hormone, progesterone, and cortisol. If estradiol, progesterone, and testosterone are replaced adequately and checked by lab tests, the thyroid may be hyperfunctioning. High thyroid hormone blood levels, especially T3, cause the temperature to rise and the heart to hyperfunction. If thyroid hormone is not the problem, then cortisol may be low, as adrenal burnout can cause very high temperatures. Levels of all hormones should be checked to make sure they are in the normal biologic range.

Older women (over 70) either require very little hormone to help them feel better or will need twice as much as younger women.

Some older women do not respond to the usual dose of estrogen because they have lost receptor sites all over their bodies. When estradiol blood levels are between 60 and 250 pg/ml and a woman still has a dry vagina and hot flashes, the number of years she was without estrogen and testosterone before replacement began should be considered in dosing. Also, blood levels quite a bit higher than normal should be considered.

THYROID HORMONE REPLACEMENT: TROUBLESHOOTING

Thyroid hormone is necessary in every system of the body. It orchestrates hormonal balance and is the "thermostat" that regulates the use of calories and modulates weight, temperature, heart rate, blood pressure, use of cholesterol, bowel movements, blood flow to the skin, and almost every enzymatic function of the body.

We must treat low thyroid hormone levels as well as other hormones that decrease as we age, such as cortisol and growth hormone, to maintain health. Thyroid hormones decrease as we age: T4 decreases 10 to 20 percent between the ages of 25 and 75, and T3 decreases by 25 percent during the same time frame.

The reality is that we are warm-blooded for a reason. Our body temperature, between 98.0 and 98.9 degrees, allows all of our enzymes to work. Without thyroid hormone we are too "cold" for metabolism and cannot burn calories, repair cells, or function optimally.

Treatment for low thyroid hormone does not resolve symptoms

Many men and women who take thyroid hormone replacement do not rid themselves of the symptoms of low thyroid hormone for two possible reasons: they cannot absorb their oral medication because they take medications that impair such absorption, or they cannot metabolize the inactive thyroid hormone, T4, into the active form, T3.

If the blood levels of T3 and T4 are both low, a diagnosis of malabsorption (poor absorption) can be made. Either a medication is blocking absorption or an untreated disease of the intestines, such as Crohn's disease, is preventing the absorption of thyroid hormone and other medications taken orally. Treatment includes changing the medication or treating the illnesses preventing the absorption.

The second reason for thyroid hormone medication failing to resolve symptoms is a genetic defect in many women (and some men) causing them to be unable to transform T4 (the inactive form of thyroid hormone) into active T3 in the cells. This problem becomes more severe with age, so when women are given medication for low thyroid hormone that consists of only T4 (Synthroid, levothyroxine, or Levoxyl), they absorb the medicine but it does no good because they cannot convert T4 into T3.

Treatment for this issue is solved by one of three interventions: add another drug that is pure T3, Cytomel (liothyronine); add bio-identical T3 in oral form plus T4; or change thyroid medications to the most efficient and least expensive replacement of both thyroid hormones, Armour Thyroid (T4 and T3 from pig thyroid). The latter allows for good absorption, inexpensive natural thyroid hormone replacement, once-a-day dosing, and efficient resolution of symptoms.

Troubleshooting thyroid medications' common side effects

The most common side effect of any thyroid hormone replacement is rapid heart rate, with or without anxiety. This is dose dependent and often goes away when dosage is decreased. If it persists, the doctor should try changing the type of thyroid hormone.

This side effect is only that; it should not be confused with evidence that the dose is more than a woman needs. Fast heart rate and anxiety are caused by stimulation of the adrenergic nerves that stimulate secretion of adrenaline and increase stimulation of the heart rate. Often a woman has this side effect but still is not getting enough thyroid hormone to keep her body warm and working efficiently. In that case it is not appropriate to settle for underdosing, but she should try every other form of thyroid medication, as well as take a thyroid hormone supplement with kelp (iodine).

When you can't tolerate thyroid hormone replacement

Cortisol deficiency causes a patient with hypothyroidism to be unable to tolerate thyroid medicine. When a very low dose of thyroid hormone replacement of any kind causes signs and symptoms of hyperthyroidism, cortisol levels should be evaluated and cortisol replaced if it is low before beginning thyroid medication again.

Iodine is necessary for thyroid function.

Iodine is essential to thyroid gland function, and women who live in the Midwest often have iodine deficiencies because there is very little or no iodine in the water or ground. Any woman living anywhere can have thyroid hormone deficiency now because we fluoridate water, which displaces iodine, and our water becomes noniodized. Our low-salt diets and the use of noniodized salt can also cause low iodine levels.

Women need more iodine than men because iodine concentrates in the breasts, and deficiencies begin during the adolescent years when women's breasts begin to grow. Often there is not enough iodine for both the breasts and thyroid, so we often see low thyroid hormone at this time in a woman's life. Fibrous breast cysts are one sign of iodine deficiency.

Iodine is necessary for T4 to convert to T3. To supplement iodine and support thyroid activity, a daily dose of dried (not roasted) kelp will improve iodine levels. Other supplements that have kelp in them, or the supplement Iodoral (taken once per day for the first month and then a half dose per day thereafter), actually cause the thyroid gland to slow down and stop! It is best to follow the instructions for dosage on supplements and not to overdose.

The environment changes the necessary dose of thyroid hormone replacement.

When the thyroid is working properly, it increases production when our bodies are exposed to certain circumstances. The body passes this information to the brain, and the pituitary stimulates the thyroid to work at a higher rate. When taking thyroid hormone we must have our dose adjusted because our bodies are not able to stimulate the level of thyroid hormone while we are taking thyroid supplementation.

Conditions that require more thyroid hormone replacement—a 5 to 20 percent increase:

- Beta blockers
- Cold weather
- Excessive exercise
- High altitudes
- High-protein diet
- Low-calorie diet
- Sleep deprivation

How to alter thyroid hormone levels with other hormones:

- Thyroid function is stimulated by growth hormone, testosterone, melatonin, progesterone, and cortisol.
- Thyroid function is inhibited by oral estrogen and high doses of cortisol medications.

Normal levels for thyroid hormone have changed through research and have been found to be gender specific. Laboratory tests by Quest Diagnostics and LabCorp rarely apply these new normal values, however, which results in women being judged based on the normal for men, and therefore frequently not treated or undertreated.

Normal Thyroid Hormone Levels (Female):

TSH (thyroid-stimulating hormone): 0.2–2.5 microunits/ml
T4 and T3 are the same as male normals

If your TSH is above 2.5 and you have symptoms of hypothyroidism, replacement with thyroid hormone is indicated.

APPENDIX B

Glossary

Ablation	Removal or destruction of a tissue or the destruction of its function
ACTH	Adrenocorticotropic hormone: hormone that stimulates the adrenal gland from the pituitary gland
Adrenal gland	A gland responsible for controlling balance of various hormones and chemicals, conversion of carbohydrates into energy, reaction to stress, balance of potassium and sodium, and sexual development
Alzheimer's disease	A progressive and disabling disease of the brain, appearing more often in women from 40 to 60 years old than it does in men. It is characterized by loss of memory and intellectual function. It is caused by inflammatory deposits of protein on the neurons of the brain.
Androstenedione	A type of androgen produced by the adrenal glands that is partially transformed by the body into testosterone
Anorgasmia	The inability to achieve orgasm
Anovulation	Lack of ovulation
Arrhythmia	Loss of rhythm or irregular rhythm of the heartbeat
ASA	Acetylsalicylic acid—aspirin
Atherosclerosis	The accumulation of plaque on the arteries
Atrophy	The wasting away of tissue or organ
Autoimmune disease	A disorder wherein the immune system attacks the body
Axillary lymph nodes	Lymph nodes under the armpit
Blood-brain barrier	A membrane between circulating blood and the brain that prevents damaging substances from reaching the brain and spinal fluid

Buccal	The area of the cheek
Chelation therapy	A chemical process in which a synthetic solution is injected into the bloodstream to remove heavy metals and/or minerals from the body
Chronic illness	An ongoing, long-lasting health problem
Collagen	A protein found in the connective tissues of the skin, bones, ligaments, and cartilage
Compounded medicine	A medication made from scratch in a compounding pharmacy
Conjugated	Paired or joined together
Contraindication	Any condition or circumstance that makes an otherwise effective therapy inappropriate
Corpus luteum	The mass of cells that form once the egg has been released from the ovary
Cortisol	A hormone produced by the adrenal gland that responds to stress
Cystocele	A hernia in the vagina that contains the bladder and protrudes into the vagina
Deep venous thrombosis (DVT)	A blood clot in a vein that has the potential of traveling to the heart and lungs
Dihydrotestosterone (DHT)	A metabolite of testosterone that affects the prostate gland, testes, hair follicles, and adrenal glands
Dilation and curettage (D&C)	The dilation of the cervical canal and scraping of tissue from the uterus
Echocardiogram	An ultrasound image of the beating heart and structures within it
Edema	The accumulation of fluid in the tissues, resulting in swelling
Embolism	Solid, liquid, or gaseous matter obstructing a blood vessel
Endocrine gland	A gland that secretes hormones into the bloodstream, not through a duct; e.g., pituitary gland, pancreas, ovaries, testes, thyroid gland, parathyroid gland, adrenal glands
Endocrinology	The study of hormones
Endometrial	Pertaining to the lining of the uterus
Endometriosis	Bits of uterine tissue that have migrated and adhered to other parts of the pelvic cavity
Epstein-Barr virus	The virus that causes mononucleosis and one of the causes of chronic fatigue

Estriol	Estrogen produced from the placenta in pregnancy, as well as a metabolite of estradiol and estrone
Estrone	The "bad" or "old lady" estrogen hormone produced in the adrenal gland; called that because it occurs only when testosterone decreases and we begin to age under the influence of this estrogen
Fibroid	A benign fibrous tumor, most often found in the uterus
First-pass effect	When a medication is taken through the stomach, processed through the liver, and changed into different metabolites that act differently from the drug taken
Free hormone	The active form of the hormone that is "free" of binding, which makes it able to stimulate target cells
FSH (follicle-stimulating hormone)	A hormone from the pituitary that stimulates the ovary with pulses that prompt it to make estradiol and mature an egg
Gold therapy	Salts used to treat rheumatoid arthritis, lupus, and some cancers
Granuloma	A growth or tumor, usually of lymph and epithelial cells
Growth hormone (also HGH, somatotropin)	A pituitary hormone that increases growth early in life and decreases with age and weight gain. Exercise, sleep, and lean body mass increase production of GH.
HbA1c (hemaglobin A1c)	Blood glucose attaches irreversibly to the beta chain of hemoglobin and reflects the average blood glucose over the past 6 to 12 weeks. Normal is <5.7.
High cardiac CRP (C-reactive protein) Inflammation	A protein that is produced by the body during the process of inflammation. High CRP is related to cardiac disease, obesity, and autoimmune disorders.
Hirsutism	Excessive hair growth, especially on the face, chest, and abdomen
Hormone	A regulatory liquid produced by a gland and transported in the bloodstream, with the purpose of stimulating specific cells into action
Hormone metabolite	A "piece" or by-product of a hormone that is produced during the degradation of an original hormone by the liver. Metabolites have different effects than the original hormone.
Hyperlipidemia	An excessive quantity of fat in the blood
Hyperplasia	An excessive number of normal cells
Hypertension, hypertensive	High blood pressure, above 140 over 90
Hyperthyroidism	Excessive thyroid hormone
Hypoglycemia	A low level of glucose in the blood
Hypoparathyroidism	Insufficient parathyroid hormone

Hypothyroidism	Insufficient thyroid hormone
Impingement	Being pinched or cut off
Insomnia	Poor or nonrestful sleep characterized by difficulty falling asleep, lack of dreaming or REM sleep, waking in the early morning hours, and/or difficulty falling back to sleep
Insulin resistance	A condition in which the cells have a diminished ability to respond to the action of insulin, resulting in the secretion of more insulin. It is thought to be a marker that precedes diabetes and can be tied to high blood pressure, abnormal cholesterol levels, heart disease, obesity, and kidney damage.
Intramuscular	Within or into the muscles
Keloid	A raised, firm, thick scar
Labile	Unstable or changeable
LH (luteinizing hormone)	A hormone from the pituitary that stimulates the ovary and peaks before ovulation, stimulating ovulation, a surge of testosterone, and progesterone production
Libido	All the components of a person's sex drive that makes them want to have sex, including sexual thoughts or fantasies, sexual attraction, and desire to have sex
Lipid	Fat or fatlike substances
Malaise	Illness or a general feeling of discomfort
Metabolism	Level of energy expenditure
Metabolite	A product of metabolism
Migraine	A severe headache characterized by sensitivity to light, disordered vision, and gastrointestinal upsets (nausea)
Morbidity	Disease, illness
Myasthenia gravis	A disease characterized by muscular weakness and increasing fatigue
Narcolepsy	A syndrome characterized by uncontrolled sleeping during the day and disrupted nighttime sleep
Neurotransmitters	Hormones in the brain that are liquid communicators; e.g., dopamine, serotonin, norepinephrine
NIH	National Institutes of Health
Norepinephrine	A hormone produced by the adrenal gland that acts as a stimulant
Osteoporosis	Thinning of the bones, especially of the vertebrae and hip
OTC	Over the counter, as medications easily located in the aisles of drug stores, grocery stores, etc.

Ovaries	Two glands in females that contain the ovum (egg) and secrete three hormones
Ovulation	The time during which the ovum (egg) ripens, erupts from the ovary, and travels through the fallopian tube into the uterus
Parenteral	A route other than oral for taking any substance into the body; e.g., intravenous, subcutaneous, vaginal
Perimenopause	The period of time near and before menopause characterized by hormonal imbalance
Pituitary	The gland in the brain that orchestrates and controls the other glands; responsible for secreting FSH, LH, ACTH, prolactin, TSH, MSH, and vasopressin
Placenta	A life support system for a baby—found only in pregnancy and made by both the uterus and the fetus—that acts as a gland, making the estrogen, estriol, and progesterone as well as androgens
Polycystic	Containing many cysts
Polycythemia	An excess of red blood cells
Polyp	A benign tumor on a stemlike structure that looks like a punching bag
Progesterone	A female hormone responsible for changes in the uterine lining in the second half of the menstrual cycle and for development of the placenta after fertilization
Progestin	A synthetic hormone similar to progesterone, with different effects and side effects throughout the body that are dissimilar to progesterone
Prolapse	Falling down or dropping of an organ or internal part; e.g., prolapsed uterus
Prophylaxis	Something used to prevent disease
Rapid eye movement sleep (REM)	Cyclic movement of the closed eyes during sleep, associated with dreaming
Receptor site	An area on a target cell wall or membrane where a hormone can attach to and activate the cell
Rectocele	Protrusion or herniation of the rectum into the vaginal wall
Serotonin	A neurologic hormone that improves mood
Sex hormone	A specialized hormone for the development of sexual characteristics (breasts, hips, pubic hair) and reproduction; e.g., estradiol, testosterone, and progesterone. They are produced in the ovaries and the testes.

Sex hormone binding globulin (SHBG)	The main protein that binds testosterone and estradiol in the blood
Spatial sense	The sense of the three-dimensional space around the body
Spontaneous fracture	A fracture occurring without obvious cause, sometimes painlessly
Stenosis	Constriction or narrowing, especially of an artery
Stimulatory hormone	A hormone produced by the pituitary gland that sends activation messages to other glands around the body to cause them to produce specific hormones. Some of them have "SH" in their names, such as FSH and TSH.
Subdermal	Below the skin, in the fat layer
Sublingual	Beneath the tongue
Suppository	A semisolid substance inserted into the rectum or vagina that dissolves and allows a medication to be absorbed by the body
Synthetic	Not found in nature or made from natural compounds, but made in the laboratory
Target cells	Cells throughout the body that have unique receptors that bind to a specific hormone and carry out the activity communicated by that hormone
TED hose	Stockings used to prevent deep venous thrombosis, skin breakdown, and worsening of varicose veins
Thrombocytosis	Increase in the number of blood platelets
Thyroid gland	The gland responsible for controlling metabolism, chemical reactions in the body, and the amount of calcium and cholesterol in the blood
Transdermal	Through or via the skin
Turgor	Distension or swelling
Ultrasound	Images taken by a machine that uses inaudible sound waves to view organs and tissues
Vascular disease	A disease or disorder of the blood circulatory system
Vulva	Female exterior anatomy pertaining to the labia, clitoris, and vagina
WHI	A Women's Health Initiative study on the use of hormone replacement therapy by menopausal women, 2002

APPENDIX C

List of Medications That May Be Replaced by Hormone Replacement

Kathy has found that many of her patients are able to discontinue medications they took before starting their bio-identical replacement hormones. Hormone replacement treats the cause of the condition or disease, so the symptomatic treatment often can be discontinued after 6 to 12 months of treatment. It is not always the case, but she finds that most people regain their health after replacement of their missing hormones and are able to stop taking multiple medications for symptoms that are relieved after replacement of testosterone.

Medications That Are Commonly Discontinued with the Addition of Testosterone (T), Estrogen (E), or Thyroid Hormone (TH)

Medical Illness	Medication Replaced by T, E, or TH	How T, E, and TH Work on the Problem
Antianxiety medications	Xanax, Ativan, etc.	T and E decrease anxiety
Antibiotics for bladder infections	Septra, Bactrim, Cipro, Macrobid	T and E decrease the frequency of bladder infections
Antidepressants	Prozac, Wellbutrin, Celexa, Lexapro, Cymbalta, etc.	T and TH improve mood and stability of mood

Antifungals for yeast infection	Diflucan, Monistat, Nystatin	T thickens the lining of the vagina and balances the pH of the vagina and GI tract
Antihypertensives	Medication for low blood pressure	T decreases fat, increases lean body mass, and relaxes blood vessels
Cholesterol-lowering medications	All statin drugs, e.g., Lipitor, simvastatin	T and TH lower total cholesterol
Diabetes	Metformin, rosiglitiazone, all the sulfonylureas and Biguanides	T and E improve insulin resistance and promote fat loss; TH helps weight loss
Drugs for autoimmune diseases	Cymbalta, Remicade, Humira, Plaquenil, Azulfidine, Enbrel	T decreases inflammation and the autoimmune response
Drugs for chronic pain	Hydrocodone, codeine, Ultram, etc.	T increases pain threshold
Hair loss	Propecia, minoxidil	E and TH increase hair growth
Heart failure	Make all drugs work better but they are required	T and TH increase the strength of the heart muscle
Migraine medications	Axert, Imitrex, Ergotamine, Fioricet, Frova, Maxalt, and all triptans	T decreases the incidence and severity of migraine headaches
Osteoporosis	Bisphosphonates such as Fosamax, Actonel, Boniva	T and E grow bone back to normal strength in less time than any bisphosphonate
Swelling	All diuretics	T and TH decrease extracellular water, swelling
Vaginal dryness	Lubricants, vaginal creams	T or E relieves vaginal dryness and painful intercourse

BIBLIOGRAPHY

"A Practical Approach to the Patient with Subclinical Hypothyroidism" in *A Clinical Conundrum: The Diagnosis and Treatment of Androgen Deficiency in Older Men.* Mayo Clinic Communiqué, September 2007: 5–6.

Ackerman, Lindsey S. "Sex Hormones and the Genesis of Autoimmunity." *The Journal of the American Medical Association Dermatology* 142, no. 3, 371.

Affinito, P., S. Palomba, M. Bonifacio et al. "Effects of Hormonal Replacement Therapy in Postmenopausal Hypertensive Patients." *Maturitas* 40, no. 1 (October 31, 2001): 75–83.

Akhrass, F., A. Evans, W. Yue et al. "Hormone Replacement Therapy Is Associated with Less Coronary Atherosclerosis in Postmenopausal Women." *The Journal of Clinical Endocrinology & Metabolism* 88 (2003): 5611–14.

Alexander, J. L., and K. Kotz. "Libido/Sexuality and the Menopause." *Menopause and Sexuality* (August 2003): 11–15.

Alexander, J. L., K. Kotz, L. Dennerstein et al. "The Systemic Nature of Sexual Functioning in the Postmenopausal Woman: Crossroads of Psychiatry and Gynecology." *Primary Psychiatry* 10, no. 12 (December 2003): 53–57.

American College of Obstetricians and Gynecologists. "Androgen Treatment of Decreased Libido." *American Journal of Obstetrics & Gynecology,* Committee Opinion, no. 244 (November 2000): 1–2.

American College of Obstetricians and Gynecologists. "Postmenopausal Estrogen Therapy: Route of Administration and Risk of Venous Embolism." *American Journal of Obstetrics & Gynecology,* Committee Opinion, no. 556 (April 2013).

Amory, J., N. Watts, K. Easley et al. "Exogenous Testosterone or Testosterone with Finasteride Increases Bone Mineral Density in Older Men with Low Serum Testosterone." *The Journal of Clinical Endocrinology & Metabolism* 89, no. 2 (2004): 503–10.

Anawalt, Bradley D. "Androgens in Health and Disease" in *Contemporary Endocrinology: Androgens in Health and Disease,* edited by C. Bagatell and W. J. Bremner. Totowa, NJ: Humana Press, 2001.

"Androgen Deficiency and the Metabolic Syndrome." *Endocrine News.* (March 2006): 7.

Ansell, Benjamin J. "The Metabolic Syndrome in Postmenopausal Women." *Contemporary OB/GYN* (May 2003): 77–83.

Archer, David F. "Estradiol Gel: A New Option in Hormone Replacement Therapy." *OBG Management* (September 2004): 46–64.

————. "Hormone Therapy and Breast Cancer: Issues in Counseling Women." *Menopausal Medicine* 13, no. 3 (Winter 2005): 5–11.

Arem, Ridha. *The Thyroid Solution.* New York: Ballantine, 1999.

Bachmann, G., J. Bancroft, G. Braunstein et al. "Female Androgen Insufficiency." *Fertility and Sterility* 77 (2002): 660–65.

Bachmann, Gloria A. "Strategies for Recognition and Management of Sexual Dysfunction in Menopausal Women." *Contemporary OB/GYN Supplement* (September 2004): 4–25.

Bachmann, Gloria, John E. Buster, and James Simon. "The Safety and Efficacy of Testosterone in Menopausal Women." *Contemporary OB/GYN* (September 2004): 2–26.

Barlow, D., H. Abdalla, A. Roberts et al. "Long-Term Hormone Implant Therapy—Hormonal and Clinical Effects." *Obstetrics & Gynecology* 67, no. 3 (March 1986): 321–25.

Beral, V. "Timing of Hormone Therapy Reduced Breast Cancer Risk." *National Cancer Institute* 103 (2011): 1–10.

Berman, Laura, and Jennifer Berman. *Secrets of the Sexually Satisfied Woman.* New York: Hyperion, 2005.

Bikman, B., D. Zheng, W. Pories et al. "Mechanism for Improved Insulin Sensitivity after Gastric Bypass Surgery." *The Journal of Clinical Endocrinology & Metabolism* (December 2008): 4656–61.

Boccardi, M. et al. "Effects of Hormone Therapy on Brain Morphology of Healthy Postmenopausal Women." *Menopause* (July/August 2006): 584–91.

Bondy, Carolyn A. "Androgens and Breast Cancer Risk." *Menopause Management* (March/April 2005): 33–35.

Braunstein, Glenn D. "Androgen Insufficiency in Women: Summary of Critical Issues." *Fertility and Sterility* 77, no. S4 (April 2002): S94–S99.

Brincat, M., A. Magos, J. W. Studd et al. "Subcutaneous Hormone Implants for the Control of Climacteric Symptoms." *The Lancet* (January 7, 1984): 16–18.

Bruining, Kersti. "Managing Migraine: A Women's Health Issue." *Sexuality, Reproduction, and Menopause* 2, no. 4 (December 2004): 209–12.

Burger, Henry G. "Androgen Production in Women." *Fertility and Sterility* 77, no. S. 4 (April 2002): S3–S5.

Buster, John E. "Aging, Androgens, and Female Sexual Desire: Can We Restore What Time Takes Away?" *Sexuality, Reproduction, and Menopause* 3, no.1 (May 2005): 3–17.

———. "Hypoactive Sexual Desire Disorder in Postmenopausal Women: Hormonal Aspects." *OBG Management* (March 2005): 10–14.

Buster, J., S. Kingsberg, O. Aguirre et al. "Testosterone Patch for Low Sexual Desire in Surgically Menopausal Women: A Randomized Trial." *Journal of the American College of Obstetricians and Gynecologists* 105, no. 5, Part 1 (May 2005): 944–52.

Buysse, Daniel J., Anne Germain, and Douglas E. Moul. "Diagnosis, Epidemiology, and Consequences of Insomnia." *Primary Psychiatry* (August 2005): 37–50.

Cardozo, L., D. Gibb, S. Tuck et al. "The Effects of Subcutaneous Hormone Implants During the Climacteric." *Elsevier Science Publishers B.V.* (1984): 177–84.

Carr, Molly C. "The Emergence of the Metabolic Syndrome with Menopause." *The Journal of Clinical Endocrinology & Metabolism* 88, no. 6 (2003): 2404.

Chalas, Eva. "Ovaries, Estrogen and Longevity." *Obstetrics & Gynecology* 121, no. 4 (April 2013): 701–702.

Chang, Jeffrey, Kathryn A. Martin, and Robert A. Vigersky. "The Hormone Foundation's Patient Guide to the Evaluation and Treatment of Hirsutism in Premenopausal Women." *The Journal of Clinical Endocrinology & Metabolism* 92, no. 4 (April 2008).

Chappell, M., B. Westwood, L. Yamaleyava et al. "Differential Effects of Sex Steroids in Young and Aged Female mRen2.Lewis Rats: A Model of Estrogen and Salt-Sensitive Hypertension." *Gender Medicine* 5, no. SA (2009): S65–S66.

Cintolot, Rebekah. "Letrozole Reduces Distant Recurrence in Hormone Receptor-Positive Breast Cancer." *HemOnc Today* (February 1, 2006): 34.

"Common Questions About Blood Clotting Disorders." *Contemporary OB/GYN* 47, no. 10 (October 2002): 79–80.

Davis, Susan R. "Testosterone Enhances Estradiol's Effects on Postmenopausal Bone Density and Sexuality." *Maturitis* 21, no. 3 (1995): 227–36.

Davison, S., R. Bell, S. Donath et al. "Androgen Levels in Adult Females: Changes with Age, Menopause, and Oophorectomy." *The Journal of Clinical Endocrinology & Metabolism* 90, no. 7 (2005): 3847–53.

Dimitrakakis, Constantine, Jian Zhou, and Carolyn A. Bondy. "Androgens and Mammary Growth and Neoplasia." *Fertility and Sterility* 77, no. S4 (April 2002): S26–S31.

Evangelista, Odette, and Mary Ann McLaughlin. "Review of Cardiovascular Risk Factors in Women." *Gender Medicine* 6, theme issue (2009): 17–30.

Farish, E., C. Fletcher, D. Hart et al. "The Effects of Hormone Implants on Serum Lipoproteins and Steroid Hormones in Bilaterally Oophorectomised Women." *Acta Endocrinologica* 106, no. 1 (1984): 116–20.

Fenichel, Rebecca, and Terry F. Davies. "When Should You Screen for and Treat Mild Hypothyroidism?" *Contemporary OB/GYN* 51, no. 1 (January 2006): 46–53.

Freeman, Sarah B. "Menopause without HRT: Complementary Therapies." *Contemporary Nurse Practitioner,* January/February 1995: 40–49.

Geer, Eliza B., and Wei Shen. "Gender Differences in Insulin Resistance, Body Composition, and Gender Medicine." *Gender Medicine* 6, supplement issue (2009): 60–75.

Genazzani, Andrea et al. "Women's Sexuality After Menopause: What Role for Androgens?" *Sexuality, Reproduction and Menopause* 2, no. 4 (December 2004): 204–208.

Goldstein, Steven R. "Estrogen Deficiency During Menopause: 1. Its Role in the Metabolic Syndrome." *OBG Management,* no. S1 (May 2005): S1–S12.

Gordon, Mark. *The Clinical Application of Interventional Endocrinology.* Beverly Hills, CA: Phoenix Books, Inc., 2008.

Gorman, Christine, and Alice Park. "The New Science of Headaches." *Time* (May 8, 2007): 76–82.

Gracia, C., E. Freeman, M. Sammel et al. "Hormones and Sexuality During Transition to Menopause." *Obstetrics & Gynecology* 109, no. 4 (April 2007): 831–32.

Granberg, S., K. Eurenius, R. Lindgren et al. "The Effects of Oral Estriol on the Endometrium in Postmenopausal Women." *Maturitas* 42, no. 2 (June 25, 2002): 149–56.

Greenblatt, Robert B., and Roland R Suran. "Indications for Hormonal Pellets in the Therapy of Endocrine and Gynecologic Disorders." *American Journal of Obstetrics & Gynecology,* 57 (1949): 294–3301.

Greer, Ian. "Venous Thromboembolism and Anticoagulant Therapy in Pregnancy." *Gender Medicine* 2, no. SA (2005): S10–S17.

Guzick, David S. "Can Postmenopausal Women Patch Up Their Sex Lives with Testosterone?" *Journal of the American College of Obstetricians and Gynecologists,* 105, no. 5, Part 1 (May 2005): 938.

Haigh, Christen. "Abnormal IR Can Precipitate Pathological Conditions." *Endocrine Today* (January 2008): 32.

Haiken, M. et al. "Why Do I Feel So Premenstrual, Lethargic, Moody, Tired, Depressed, Forgetful, Fat, Bloated? It Could Be Your Thyroid." *Health* (June 2006): 102–107.

Hajszan, T., N. MacLusky, J. Johansen et al. "Effects of Androgens and Estradiol on Spine Synapse Formation in the Prefrontal Cortex of Normal and Testicular Feminization Mutant Male Rats." *Endocrinology* 148, no. 5 (May 2007): 963–67.

Hall, S., G. Esche, A. Araujo et al. "Correlates of Low Testosterone and Symptomatic Androgen Deficiency in a Population-Based Sample." *The Journal of Clinical Endocrinology & Metabolism* 93, no. 10 (October 2008): 3870–77.

Hamilton, T., S. Davis, L. Onstad et al. "Thyrotropin Levels in a Population with No Clinical, Autoantibody, or Ultrasonographic Evidence of Thyroid Disease: Implications for the Diagnosis of Subclinical Hypothyroidism." *The Journal of Clinical Endocrinology & Metabolism* 93, no. 4 (April 2008): 1224–30.

Harzog, Beverly Blair. "Have Sex, Beat Migraines?" *Healthy Body* (March 2007): 82.

Hertoghe, Thierry. *The Hormone Handbook*. Luxemburg: International Medical Book, 2010.

Hoeger, Kathleen M. "Polycystic Ovary Syndrome, Inflammation, and Statins: Do We Have the Right Target?" *The Journal of Clinical Endocrinology & Metabolism* 94, no. 1 (January 2009): 35–37.

Holland, E., A. Leather, and J. Studd. "The Effects of 25-mg Percutaneous Estradiol Implants on the Bone Mass of Postmenopausal Women." *Obstetrics & Gynecology* 83, no. 1 (January 1994): 43–46.

Hollingsworth, Margarita, and Jennifer Berman. "The Role of Androgens in Female Sexual Dysfunction." *Sexuality, Reproduction, and Menopause* 4, no. 1 (May 2006): 27–32.

Honma, N., K. Takubo, M. Sawabe et al. "Estrogen-Metabolizing Enzymes in Breast Cancer from Women over the Age of 80 Years." *The Journal of Clinical Endocrinology & Metabolism* (2006): 607–13.

Hugo, E., D. Borcherding, K. Gersin et al. "Prolactin Release by Adipose Explants, Primary Adipocytes, and LS14 Adipocytes." *Journal of Clinical Endocrinology & Metabolism* 93, no. 10 (October 2008): 4006–12.

Hutchinson, Susan. "Menstrual Migraine: The Role of Hormonal Management." *The Female Patient* 32, (March 2007) 49–54.

———. "The Stages of a Woman's Life." *ACHE American Council for Headache Education* 16, no. 2 (Fall 2005): 1–2.

Jacobs, H. S., J. D. Hutton, M. A. F. Murray, and V. H. T. James. "Plasma Hormone Profiles in Post-Menopausal Women Before and During Oestrogen Therapy." *British Journal of Obstetrics and Gynecology* 84, no. 4 (April 1977): 314.

Jancin, Bruce. "Study: HT Cuts Breast Cancer Mortality 47%." *ObGynNews* (January 15, 2009): 3.

Janssen, Jennifer S., and M. McDermott. "Update on Benign Thyroid Disorders in Women." *The Female Patient* 32 (January 2007): 49–54.

Jones, Stephen C. "Subcutaneous Estrogen Replacement Therapy." *The Journal of Reproductive Medicine* 49, no. 3 (March 2004): 139–42.

King, Steven R., and D. Lamb. "Why We Lose Interest in Sex: Do Neurosteroids Play a Role?" *Sexuality, Reproduction and Menopause* 4, no. 1 (May 2006): 20–26.

Kingsberg, Sheryl A., John E. Buster, and Jan Shifren. "Menopause and Sexual Health: The Role of Testosterone." *OBG Management,* Supplement (March 2005): 3–21.

Kirn, Timothy F. "HT Patch Has Less Impact on Coagulation Factors." *Journal Watch* 24, no. 10 (May 15, 2004): 8a–8d.

Komaroff, Anthony L. "Fatigue and Chronic Fatigue Syndrome" in *Primary Care of Women,* edited by K. J. Karlson and S. A. Eisenstat, St. Louis, MO: Mosby, 2002: 615–623.

Komisaruk, Barry, Carlos Berg-Flores, and Beverly Whipple. *The Science of Orgasm.* Baltimore, MD: Johns Hopkins University Press, 2006.

Kratzert, Kristen J., and Anne M. Fontana. "The Use of Botanicals for the Treatment of Menopausal Symptoms: Weeds or Wonders?" *Menopause Management* (May/June 2005): 9–13.

Krebs, E., K. Ensrud, R. MacDonald et al. "Phytoestrogens for Treatment of Menopausal Symptoms: A Systematic Review." *The American College of Obstetricians and Gynecologists* 104, no. 4 (October 2004): 824–36.

Kremer, R., P. Campbell, T. Reinhardt et al. "Vitamin D Status and Its Relationship to Body Fat, Final Height, and Peak Bone Mass in Young Women." *The Journal of Clinical Endocrinology and Metabolism* 94, no. 1 (January 2009): 67–73.

Krychman, Michael L. "Female Sexual Dysfunction." *The Female Patient* 32 (January 2007): 47–48.

Krychman, Michael L., and Edith A. Perez. "Aromatase Inhibitors in Early Breast Cancer: Recent Adjuvant Trial Results in the Management of Breast Cancer: Clinical Implications of Aromatase Inhibitors." *The Female Patient* 1, no. 3 (December 2004): 2–10.

Lake, Alvin E., III, "Take Control of Headache: The Stress Connection." American Council for Headache Education: 1–3.

Lamberts, Steven W. J. "Endocrinology and Aging" in *Williams Textbook of Endocrinology, 12th Edition.* Kenneth S. Polonsky, P. Reed Larsen, and Henry M. Kronenberg, eds. Philadelphia, PA: Elsevier Saunders, 2011.

Langer, Robert D. "Strategies to Optimize the Safety of Hormone Therapy." *OBG Management* (November 2004): 10–14.

Langer, R., J. Simon et al. "Nonoral Options in Hormone Therapy: Lotions, Rings, and Other Things." *OBG Management* (November 2004): S2–S19.

Lewis, Jay. "Androgen Deficiency Can Cause Sexual Dysfunction." *Endocrine Today* (July 2006): 57.

Lobo, R. A. "Menopause and Sexuality: The Impact of Hormones." *Contemporary OB/GYN* Supplement (August 2003): S3–S8.

———. "The Physiology of Androgens after Menopause: What Constitutes Androgen Deficiency? Menopause and Sexuality: The Impact of Hormones." *Contemporary OB/GYN* (April 2005): 3–5.

Lobo, R. A. et al. "Considerations in Evaluating, Diagnosing, and Treating HSDD in Postmenopausal Women." *Contemporary OB/GYN* Supplement (April 2005): 4–12.

Lobo, R., C. March, U. Goebelsmann et al. "Subdermal Estradiol Pellets Following Hysterectomy and Oophorectomy." *American Journal of Obstetrics & Gynecology* 138, no. 6 (November 15, 1980): 714–19.

Low, D., S. Davis, D. Keller et al. "Cutaneous and Hemodynamic Responses During Hot Flashes in Symptomatic Postmenopausal Women." *The Journal of the North American Menopause Society* 15, no. 2 (2008): 290–295.

MacGregor, A. "Migraine Associated with Menstruation." *Functional Neurology* 15, no. S3 (2000): S143–53.

Maki, Pauline M. "Effects of Hormone Therapy on Cognitive Function: State of the Science Post-WHI." *Menopause Management* (March/April 2005): 21–23.

Martin, Vince. "Hormones and Headache: A New Frontier in Migraine Research." American Council for Headache Education: 1–5.

Meeston, Cindy M. and David M. Buss. *Why Women Have Sex*. New York: Times Books, 2009.

Miller, Ellen Hirschman. "Endocrinopathies in Women: Detection and Treatment." *The Forum* 5, no. 1 (April 2007) 4–11.

Miller, E. H. et al. "Sleep Disorders and Women." *Clinical Cornerstone* 6, no. S1B (2004): S1–S32.

Miller, K., W. Rosner, L. Hang et al. "Measurement of Free Testosterone in Normal Women and Women with Androgen Deficiency: Comparison of Methods." *The Journal of Endocrinology & Metabolism* 89, no. 2 (2004): 525–33.

Mishell, Daniel R. "A Clinical Study of Estrogenic Therapy with Pellet Implantation." *American Journal of Obstetrics & Gynecology* 41 (1941): 1009–17.

Mitwally, Mohamed F. M., and Robert F. Casper. "Aromatase Inhibitors, A New Option for Inducing Ovulation." *OBG Management* (January 2008): 57–74.

Mitwally, Mohamed F. M., Robert F. Casper, and Michael P. Diamond. "Clinical Uses of Aromatase Inhibitors: Beyond Breast Cancer." *The Female Patient* 31 (October 2006) 50–58.

Munir, Jawad, and Stanley J. Birge. "Vitamin D Deficiency in Pre- and Postmenopausal Women." *Menopause Management* (September/October 2008): 10–15.

Nelson, Erik R., and Hamid R. Habibi. "Functional Significance of Nuclear Estrogen Receptor Subtypes in the Liver of Goldfish." *General Endocrinology* (April 2010): 1668.

Nelson, Miriam E. "Strength Training for the Midlife Woman." *Menopause Management* (September/ October 2000): 17–23.

Neubauer, David, Milton K. Erman, and Phyllis Zee. "New Perspectives in the Diagnosis and Management of Insomnia." *Primary Psychiatry* Supplement 2 (December 2008).

Notelovitz, Morris. "Androgens and Hormonal Treatment Options." *Sexuality: The Impact of Hormones* (August 2003): 16–20.

———. "Androgen Effects on Bone and Muscle." *Fertility and Sterility* 77, no. S4 (April 2002): S34–S35.

Notelovitz, M., M. Johnson, S. Smith et al. "Metabolic and Hormonal Effects of 2-mg and 50-mg 17 B-Estradiol Implants in Surgically Menopausal Women." *Obstetrics & Gynecology* 70, no. 5 (November 1987): 749–54.

Parmet, Sharon, Cassio Lynm, and Richard M. Glass. "Genetics and Breast Cancer." *The Journal of the American Medical Association* 292, no. 4 (July 28, 2004): 522.

Payne, Sarah. "Sex, Gender, and Irritable Bowel Syndrome: Making the Connections." *Gender Medicine* 1, no. 1 (2004): 18–24.

Pilz, S., W. März, B. Wellnitz et al. "Association of Vitamin D Deficiency with Heart Failure and Sudden Cardiac Death in a Large Cross-Sectional Study of Patients Referred to Coronary Angiography." *The Journal of Clinical Endocrinology & Metabolism* 93, no. 10 (October 2008): 3927–35.

Pingitore, A., E. Galli, A. Barison et al. "Acute Effects of Triiodothyronine (T3) Replacement Therapy in Patients with Chronic Heart Failure and Low-T3 Syndrome: A Randomized, Placebo-Controlled Study." *The Journal of Clinical Endocrinology & Metabolism* 93, no. 4 (April 2008): 1351–58.

Polan, Mary Lake. "Androgens in Women: To Replace or Not?" *OBG Management* (May 2007): 72–81.

Prandoni, Paolo. "Venous Thromboembolism Risk and Management in Women with Cancer and Thrombophilia." *Gender Medicine* 2, no. SA (2005): S28–S34.

Qiao, X., K. McConnell, R. Khalid et al. "Sex Steroids and Vascular Responses in Hypertension and Aging." *Gender Medicine* 5, no. SA (2008): S36–S60.

Quest Diagnostics. Clinical Focus, Rheumatoid Arthritis Laboratory Markers for Diagnosis and Prognosis. Quest Diagnostics. Test Summary, Testosterone, LC/MS/MS. (2006): http://www.questdiagnostics.com/testcenter/testguide.action?dc=CF_RheumatoidArthritis.

Radetti, G., W. Kleon, F. Buzi et al. "Thyroid Function and Structure Are Affected in Childhood Obesity." *The Journal of Clinical Endocrinology & Metabolism* 93, no. 12 (December 2008): 4749.

Rariy, C. M., S. J. Ratcliffe, R. Weinstein et al. "Higher Serum Free Testosterone Concentration in Older Women is Associated with Greater Bone Mineral Density, Lean Body Mass, and Total Fat Mass: The Cardiovascular Health Study." *The Journal of Clinical Endocrinology & Metabolism* 96, no. 4 (April 2011): 989–996.

Ratner, R. E., C. Chrostophi, B. Metzger et al. "Prevention of Diabetes in Women with a History of Gestational Diabetes: Effects of Metformin and Lifestyle Interventions." *The Journal of Clinical Endocrinology & Metabolism* 96, no. 4 (December 2008): 4774–79.

Redmond, Geoffrey P. "Thyroid Disease and Women's Health." *OBG Management* Supplement (October 2001): S3–S8.

Refetoff, MD, et al. "New Genetic Thyroid Defect Identified." *Endocrine News* (March 2007): 14–21.

Rehman, Habib, and Ewan A. Masson. "Neuroendocrinology of Female Aging." *Gender Medicine* 2, no. 1 (2005): 41–56.

Roberts, Barbara, and Paul D. Thompson. "Is There Evidence for the Evidence-Based Guidelines of Cardiovascular Disease Prevention in Women?" *Gender Medicine* 3, no. 1 (2006): 5–12.

Roby, Russell. "Treating Chronic Fatigue Syndrome in Austin." *Roby Institute* (2009): http://www.robyinstitute.com/treatments/chronic_fatigue_syndrome_cfs.htm.

Rosen, R., G. Bachmann, S. Leiblum et al. "Androgen Insufficiency in Women: The Princeton Conference." *Fertility and Sterility* 77, no. S4 (April 2002): S26–S47.

Russell, Jon. "Fibromyalgia Syndrome: New Developments in Pathophysiology and Management." *Primary Psychiatry* 13, no. 9 (2006): 38–39.

Saravanan, P., D. Simmons, R. Greenwood et al. "Partial Substitution of Thyroxine (T4) with Tri-Iodothyronine in Patients on T4 Replacement Therapy: Results of Large Community-based Randomized Controlled Trial." *The Journal of Clinical Endocrinology & Metabolism* 90, no. 2 (2005): 805.

Sarrel, Philip M. "Androgen Deficiency: Menopause and Estrogen-related Factors." *Fertility and Sterility* 77, no. S4 (April 2002): S63–S66.

Savvas, M., J. Studd, S. Norman et al. "Increase in Bone Mass After One Year of Percutaneous Oestradiol and Testosterone Implants in Post-Menopausal Women who Have Previously Received Long-Term Oral Oestrogens." *British Journal of Obstetrics and Gynecology*, 99 (September 1992): 757–60.

———. "Skeletal Effects of Oral Estrogen Compared with Subcutaneous Oestrogen and Testosterone in Postmenopausal Women." *British Medical Journal* 297, no. 30 (July 1988): 331–33.

Schierbeck, Louise Led. "Effect of Hormone Replacement Therapy on Cardiovascular Events in Recently Post-Menopausal Woman: Randomized Trial." *British Medical Journal* (2012): 345 doi: e 6409.

Schmidt, J., M. Binder, G. Demschik et al. "Treatment of Aging Skin with Topical Estrogens." *International Journal of Dermatology* 35, no. 9 (September 1996): 25 (paraphrased).

Schwartz, Erika, Kent Holtorf, and David Brownstein. "The Truth About Hormone Therapy." *Wall Street Journal,* March 16, 2009, national edition, section A17.

"Sexual Orientation Might Be Determined Before Birth." *Endocrine News,* edited by C. Kristiansen. (March 2006): 14.

Sherwin, Barbara B. "Randomized Clinical Trials of Combined Estrogen-Androgen Preparations: Effects on Sexual Functioning." *Fertility and Sterility* 77, no. S4, (April 2002): S49–S53.

Sherwin, B. B., and M. Gelfand. "The Role of Androgen in the Maintenance of Sexual Functioning in Oophorectomized Women." *Psychosomatic Medicine* 49, no. 4 (1987): 397–409.

Shifren, Jan L. "Androgen Deficiency in the Oophorectomized Woman." *Fertility and Sterility* 77, no. S4 (April 2002): S60–S62.

———. "Hypoactive Sexual Desire Disorder in Postmenopausal Women: Treatment Options." *OGB Management* (March 2005): 15–21.

Shulman, L. M., and Viveca Bhat. "Gender Differences in the Natural History and Management of Parkinson's Disease." *Menopause Management* (January/February 2007): 14–20.

Simon, James. "Differential Effects of Estrogen-Androgen and Estrogen-Only Therapy on Vasomotor Symptoms, Gonadotropin Secretion, and Endogenous Androgen Bioavailability in Postmenopausal Women." *Menopause* 6, no. 2 (1999): 138.

Simon, James A. "Emerging Treatment Strategies for Menopausal Women with HSDD: The Role of Testosterone Therapy." *Contemporary OB/GYN* (September 2004): 18–22.

Simpkins, J., P. Green, K. Gridley et al. "Role of Estrogen Replacement Therapy in Memory Enhancement and the Prevention of Neuronal Loss Associated with Alzheimer's Disease." *College Pharmacy Technical Bulletin* 1, no. 6 (September 15, 2003).

Simpson, Evan R. "Aromatization of Androgens in Women: Current Concepts and Findings." *Fertility and Sterility* 77, no. S4 (April 2002): S6–S10.

Sims, Cheryl. "Managing Migraine: A Patient's Perspective." *Headache:* 948–49.

Sites, Cynthia K., and Shauna L. McKinney. "The Metabolic Syndrome Impact on Women and Consideration for Treatment." *Menopausal Medicine* 16, no. 3 (August 2008): S1–S12.

Speroff, Leon. "Postmenopausal Hormone Therapy and the Risk of Breast Cancer: A Contrary Thought." *Menopause* 15, no. 2 (2008): 393–400.

———. "Using Aromatase Inhibitors to Treat Early Breast Cancer." *Contemporary OB/GYN* (February 2006): 60–64.

Splete, Heidi. "Anastrazole Tops Tamoxifen in Analasis of ATAC Trial." *Ob.Gyn. News* (December 2012): 3.

Stanczyk, F., D. Shoupe, V. Nunez et al. "A Randomized Comparison of Nonoral Estradiol Delivery in Postmenopausal Women." *American Journal of Obstetrics & Gynecology* 159, no. 6 (December 1988): 1540–46.

Staud, Roland, and Michael Spaeth. "Psychophysical and Neurochemical Abnormalities of Pain Processing in Fibromyalgia." *Primary Psychiatry* 15, no. 3, Supplement 2 (March 2008): 12–13.

Stefanick, M., G. Anderson, K. Margolis et al. "Effects of Conjugated Equine Estrogens on Breast Cancer and Mammography Screening in Postmenopausal Women with Hysterectomy." *The Journal of the American Medical Association* 295, no. 14 (April 12, 2006): 1647.

Steiner, A., L. Chang, J. Qing et al. "3α-Hydrozysteroid Dehydrogenase Type III Deficiency: A Novel Mechanism of Hirsutism." *The Journal of Clinical Endocrinology & Metabolism* 93, no. 4 (April 2008): 1298–1303.

Stenchever, Morton A., and Gretchen M. Lentz. "Sexual Dysfunction: A Couple Issue." *Contemporary OB/GYN* (December 2004): 30–44.

Stillman, Mark J. "Testosterone Replacement Therapy for Treatment Refractory Cluster Headache." *Headache* 46, no. 6 (June 2006): 925–33.

Studd, J. "Oestradiol and Testosterone Implants in the Treatment of Psychosexual Problems in the Postmenopausal Woman." *British Journal of Obstetrics & Gynecology* 84 (April 1977): 316–17.

Studd, J., M. Savvas, N. Waston et al. "The Relationship between Plasma Estradiol and the Increase in Bone Density in Postmenopausal Women after Treatment with Subcutaneous Hormone Implants." *American Journal of Obstetrics and Gynecology* 163, no. 5, Part 1 (November 1990): 1474–79.

Sulak, Patricia J., and Susan Rako. "Is Menstruation Necessary?" *The Female Patient* 31 (November 2006): 43–44.

Sullivan, Michele G. "HT May Benefit Postmenopausal Cognition, Memory." *Ob.Gyn. News* (August 15, 2008): 1, 6.

Szelke, E., T. Mersich, B. Szekacs et al "3. Effects of Estrogen and Progestin on the CO_2 Sensitivity of Hemispheric Cerebral Blood Volume." *Menopause* 15, no. 2 (2008): 345–51.

"Testosterone Plays an Important Role in Women's Health and Quality of Life." *Endocrine Today.* (July 2006): 56.

Thom, M. "Hormonal Profiles in Postmenopausal Women after Therapy with Subcutaneous Implants." *British Journal of Obstetrics and Gynecology* 88 (April 1981): 426–33.

Traish, A., N. Kim, K. Min et al. "Role of Androgens in Female Genital Sexual Arousal: Receptor Expression, Structure, and Function." *Fertility and Sterility* 77, no. S4 (April 2002): S11–S32.

Tutera, Gino. "Hope for HRT." *Advance for Healthy Aging* (September/October 2005): 10.

———. *You Don't Have to Live With It!* Palm Desert, CA: SottoPelle, 2003.

Utian, Wulf H. "Problems with Desire and Arousal in Surgically Menopausal Women: Advances in Assessment, Diagnosis and Treatment." *Menopause Management* 14 (2005): 10–22.

Veldhuis, J., J. Patrie, K. Brill et al. "Contributions of Gender and Systemic Estradiol and Testosterone Concentrations to Maximal Secretagogue Drive of Burst-Like Growth Hormone Secretion in Healthy Middle-Aged and Older Adults." *The Journal of Clinical Endocrinology & Metabolism* 89, no. 12 (2004): 6291–96.

Vigersky, R., A. Filmore-Nassar, A. Glass et al. "Thyrotropin Suppression by Metformin." *The Journal of Clinical Endocrinology & Metabolism* 91, no. 1 (2006): 225–27.

Villareel, Dennis T., and John O. Holloszy. "Effect of DHEA on Abdominal Fat and Insulin Action in Elderly Women and Men." *The Journal of the American Medical Association* 292, no. 18 (November 10, 2004): 2243–48.

Wang, Christina, and Ronald Swerdloff. "Androgen Pharmacology and Delivery Systems." *Androgens in Health and Disease: Contemporary Endocrinology*: 141–53.

Wayman, Erin. "Hormone Therapy: A Woman's Dilemma." *Endocrine News* (November 2012): 22–25.

Wehrmacher, William H., and Harry Messmore. "Women's Health Initiative Fundamentally Flawed." *Gender Medicine* 2 (2005): 4–6.

Weiss, Gerson. "The Perimenopausal Transition." *The Female Patient* 32 (March 2007): 50–52.

White, Perrin C. "Aldosterone: Direct Effects on and Production by the Heart." *The Journal of Clinical Endocrinology & Metabolism* 88, no. 6 (2003): 2376–83.

Wilkins, Kirsten M., and Julia K. Warnock. "Sexual Dysfunction in Older Women." *Primary Psychiatry* (March 2009): 59–65.

Wu, Olivia. "Postmenopausal Hormone Replacement Therapy and Venous Thromboembolism." *Gender Medicine* 2, no. SA (2005): S18–S27

Yacoub-Wasef, S. "Gender Differences in Systemic Lupus Erythematosus." *Gender Medicine* 1, no. 1 (2004): 12–16.

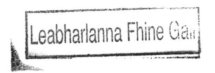

Yaffe, K., A. M. Kanaya, K. Lindquist et al. "The Metabolic Syndrome, Inflammation, and Risk of Cognitive Decline." *The Journal of the American Medical Association* (November 10, 2004): 2237.

Yang, Sarah. "Compound in Broccoli Has Immune-boosting Properties, Finds New Study." UC Berkeley Press Release (August 20, 2007).

Zandi, P. P., M. C. Carlson, B. L. Plassman et al. "Hormone Replacement Therapy and Incidence of Alzheimer's Disease in Older Women: the Cache County Study." *The Journal of the American Medical Association* 288, no. 17 (November 6, 2002): 2123–2129.

Zang, H., L. Sahlin, B. Masironi et al. "Effects of Testosterone and Estrogen Treatment on the Distribution of Sex Hormone Receptors in the Endometrium of Postmenopausal Women." *Menopause* 15, no. 2 (March/April 2008): 233–39.

Zangaria, Mary Ann E. "Sleep Disturbance in Older Women." *Women's Health Ob-Gyn Edition* (January/February 2006): 23–30.

Zee, Phyllis. "The Role of Menopause." Expert Panel Supplement: An Expert Panel Review of Clinical Challenges in Primary Care, Supplement 8 (December 2008): 7–9.

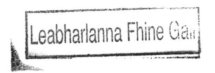

INDEX

ACKNOWLEDGMENTS

From Kathy

There is no way I can express my thanks to the people who have encouraged, helped, and motivated me to write this book. This is absolutely the most passionate work of my life, and that is saying something!

Initially, my patients were the women who requested that I write a book about the amazing healing they experienced with testosterone replacement. They have been waiting nine years, and they are my ongoing inspiration to share the "secret" of testosterone replacement. I was given the confidence that this book was needed and would be successful through God's calling. It is because of Him that I am healthy and productive, and I was called to share the treatment that had brought me, and thousands of other women, back to health and into His service. No matter what your belief is, the answer to your symptoms of aging after 40 is meant for you.

No project like writing a book is the work of one person, and my support and encouragement came from John, my husband, and Rachel, my daughter, who is now training to be a doctor of family medicine. They have only encouraged me in a project that seemed a pipe dream at the beginning and consumed my time and energy. Brett Newcomb was the answer to my prayers for someone to join me in writing and believing in this book as much as I did. He motivated me and taught me to be patient with the writing process. I am thankful to Brett's wife, Phyllis, who was our initial editor and sounding board. This book would still be pieces of paper spread across the floor of my study if Brett had not agreed to believe in the dream of this book and the importance of sharing a new synthesis of research supporting testosterone treatment for women.

The BioBalance women, my staff and colleagues, are the backbone of the work that is the foundation of my medical practice; they work with me every day in a practice that initially came under fire from the medical community. They witnessed the improvements and transformations of themselves and our patients who use Bio-Balance testosterone pellets. My team has grown over the last 11 years and now constitutes my "dream team": Susie Ahrens, RN; Sandi Redhage, NP; Laurie Sills, NP; Wendy Douglas; Angie Quigle, MA; Stacy Kaltmeyer; Kathy Miller; Joan Jackson; and my administrative assistant, Erin Camp. They have not only shared the jubilant stories of our patients but followed me to the Kansas City office every other month for ten years to care for our patients across the state. Doctors never care for their patients by themselves; they always have a dedicated and caring team they depend on, and I am grateful for the team that shares the responsibility of healing our patients.

Unless you have written a book, you probably have no idea of the difficulty and time involved in bringing it to fruition. Sadly, we all take books and the writing of them for granted and pay very little for our literary education. The daunting task truly does take the 10,000 hours that author Malcolm Gladwell claims becoming expert in your field requires.

It was not a straight path from the calling to the published book. There were several starts and stops that all contributed to the final work. Before I engaged Brett, I had writing help from Romondo Davis, my website and interactive guru, a first draft compiled by Gayle Herde, and then a second draft written with the assistance of Josiah DeBoer. I also instituted the help of a new good friend, Tim Noonan, an author by profession, and finally the man who found the wonderful publisher Hay House: Rick Broadhead, our agent.

The takeaway lesson from this journey is that if there had been no pain, there would never be jubilation in conquering the source of that pain. The task of humanity is to learn and to share our learning to help others. That can only happen if we learn to turn difficult situations inside out to bring about change. If I had not gone through a "hormone disaster," I would not have found the answer in testosterone replacement and certainly would never have written a book. The source of my motivation is both divine and very human: to change the health of women in an effective and positive way by giving them back the same hormones they enjoyed earlier in life, and in doing so, allow them to carry out their lives productively. I hope this work gives you hope and a plan to get your health and life back.

From Brett

I value beyond measure my clients who shared their stories with me and allowed me to walk the journey of therapy with them. I continue to learn from the shared experiences of the lives of my clients. For those whose stories I have used, I have altered them enough to protect your privacy. Thanks to all of you for the privilege of being able to share elements of your journey. Assuredly, any error in the presentation of these stories is mine alone. I also want to thank Dr. Maupin for inviting me to share my insights in the development of this book. I have enjoyed the process, and I have learned so much from her. I want to thank my wife, Phyllis, for all her support and help; she has always been an independent ear whose feedback and humor have kept me focused and grounded.

ABOUT THE AUTHORS

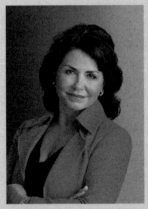

Kathy Maupin MD is a board-certified OB/GYN and founder of BioBalance Health, a practice dedicated to helping men and women in midlife who are experiencing symptoms associated with hormone deficiency. She focuses on personal care and the use of bio-identical hormone treatments to help alleviate the effects of aging. As part of her work with BioBalance Health, she co-hosts weekly video health podcasts that address current issues related to aging and relationships.

Dr Maupin is active in a variety of professional organizations including the Missouri State Medical Association, the St. Louis Metropolitan Medical Society, the St. Louis Obstetrical & Gynecological Society (for which she served as president), the American Medical Association, the American Medical Women's Association, the American Association of Women Surgeons, the American Academy of Anti-Aging Medicine, the Age Management Medicine Group and the Endocrine Society.

She is also the author of the Women's Healthcare Initiative legislation that became law in Missouri in 2000 and protects women's rights to receive care from OB/GYNs – including mammograms, bone-density testing and coverage for birth control pills – without a referral, and provides for insurance coverage for plastic surgical reconstruction for women who have had breast cancer. She is also the founder of St. Louis political action committee Physicians for Sound Healthcare Policy, and she is active in numerous charitable organizations and Greentree Community Church.

www.drkathymaupin.com
www.biobalancehealth.com

ABOUT THE AUTHORS

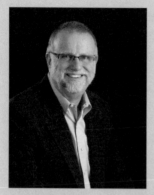

Brett Newcomb, MA, LPC has 30 years of experience in private practice as a family therapist in Missouri. He has worked with clients of all ages in myriad capacities, focusing primarily on interpersonal relationships, communication skills and family and individual problems. He has worked with Dr Maupin for years to help her patients deal with the psychological and marital ramifications of hormone imbalance and the necessary adjustments following successful treatment. In addition to his clinical experience, Brett has supervised and trained many other therapists and has taught undergraduate and graduate students at Missouri Baptist University and Webster University in St. Louis. His management experience as Webster University's World Wide Director of the Counseling Program – servicing more than 2,000 counseling students worldwide – has provided him with a broad and comprehensive perspective in the field.

In addition, Brett is the co-host with Dr Maupin of BioBalance's video health podcasts. His storytelling style weaves practical advice on current topics with engaging, entertaining and information-rich anecdotes.

www.brettnewcomb.com

If you would like more information about the recent research and science behind *The Secret Female Hormone,* or for other updated information, please visit:

thesecretfemalehormone.com

We hope you enjoyed this Hay House book. If you'd like to receive our online catalogue featuring additional information on Hay House books and products, or if you'd like to find out more about the Hay Foundation, please contact:

Hay House UK, Ltd.
Astley House, 33 Notting Hill Gate, London W11 3JQ
Phone: 0-20-3675-2450 • *Fax:* 0-20-3675-2451
www.hayhouse.co.uk • www.hayfoundation.org

❧

Published and distributed in the United States by:
Hay House, Inc., P.O. Box 5100, Carlsbad, CA 92018-5100
Phone: (760) 431-7695 or (800) 654-5126
Fax: (760) 431-6948 or (800) 650-5115
www.hayhouse.com®

Published and distributed in Australia by: Hay House Australia Pty. Ltd., 18/36 Ralph St., Alexandria NSW 2015 • *Phone:* 612-9669-4299 • *Fax:* 612-9669-4144 • www.hayhouse.com.au

Published and distributed in the Republic of South Africa by: Hay House SA (Pty), Ltd., P.O. Box 990, Witkoppen 2068 • *Phone/Fax:* 27-11-467-8904 • www.hayhouse.co.za

Published in India by: Hay House Publishers India, Muskaan Complex, Plot No. 3, B-2, Vasant Kunj, New Delhi 110 070 • *Phone:* 91-11-4176-1620 *Fax:* 91-11-4176-1630 • www.hayhouse.co.in

Distributed in Canada by: Raincoast Books, 2440 Viking Way, Richmond, B.C. V6V 1N2 • *Phone:* 1-800-663-5714 • *Fax:* 1-800-565-3770 • www.raincoast.com

❧

Take Your Soul on a Vacation

Visit www.HealYourLife.com® to regroup, recharge, and reconnect with your own magnificence.Featuring blogs, mind-body-spirit news, and life-changing wisdom from Louise Hay and friends.

Visit www.HealYourLife.com today!

Free e-newsletters
from Hay House, the Ultimate
Resource for Inspiration

Be the first to know about Hay House's dollar deals, free downloads, special offers, affirmation cards, giveaways, contests, and more!

 Get exclusive excerpts from our latest releases and videos from *Hay House Present Moments*.

 Enjoy uplifting personal stories, how-to articles, and healing advice, along with videos and empowering quotes, within *Heal Your Life*.

 Have an inspirational story to tell and a passion for writing? Sharpen your writing skills with insider tips from *Your Writing Life*.

Sign Up Now!

Get inspired, educate yourself, get a complimentary gift, and share the wisdom!

http://www.hayhouse.com/newsletters.php

Visit www.hayhouse.com to sign up today!

  HealYourLife.com

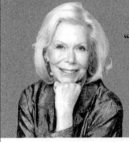
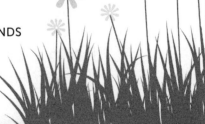